AGING ISSUES, HEALTH AND FINANCIAL ALTERNATIVES

AGEING AND MENTAL HEALTH

GLOBAL PERSPECTIVES

AGING ISSUES, HEALTH AND FINANCIAL ALTERNATIVES

Additional books in this series can be found on Nova's website under the Series tab.

Additional e-books in this series can be found on Nova's website under the e-book tab.

AGING ISSUES, HEALTH AND FINANCIAL ALTERNATIVES

AGEING AND MENTAL HEALTH

GLOBAL PERSPECTIVES

WENDY WEN LI
SHERRY M. CUMMINGS,
ILANGO PONNUSWAMI
AND
HONG-JAE PARK
EDITORS

KASSANDRA JACKSON
ASSISTANT EDITOR

nova publishers
New York

Library of Congress Cataloging-in-Publication Data

ISBN: 978-1-63484-777-3

Library of Congress Control Number: 2016932188

Published by Nova Science Publishers, Inc. † New York

CONTENTS

PREFACE

Globally, the number of elderly individuals is growing at an unprecedented rate. Currently, eleven percent of the worldwide population is 65 years and older. This number will more than double to twenty-two percent (2 billion) by 2050. As the older population continues its inexorable growth, so does the number of older adults with mental health disorders, such as Alzheimer's disease, depression, anxiety and schizophrenia. For example, the number of individuals affected by dementia worldwide is expected to double every twenty years to over 81 million by 2040. Depressive episodes in later life are also prevalent, and depression is the leading cause of disability in older adults worldwide. These mental disorders lead to increased morbidity and mortality in older adults, and often they can exact a negative toll on their family members. To respond to the ageing world, this book sets out to help researchers, policy makers, service providers, and students develop their knowledge of the issues associated with ageing and mental health throughout the world. Written by twenty-one gerontological experts from Africa, Asia, Europe, North and South America, and Oceania, this book provides an understanding of issues related to ageing and mental health from global perspectives.

In: Ageing and Mental Health: Global Perspectives
Editors: Wendy Wen Li, Sherry M. Cummings et al.
ISBN: 978-1-63484-777-3

Chapter 1

INTRODUCTION: MENTAL HEALTH IN AN AGEING WORLD

Hong-Jae Park[1,*], Wendy Wen Li[2], Sherry Cummings[3] and Ilango Ponnuswami[4]

[1]The University of Auckland, Auckland, New Zealand
[2]James Cook University, Queensland, Australia
[3]The University of Tennessee, Knoxville, Tennessee, US
[4]Bharathidasan University, Tiruchirappalli, India

ABSTRACT

This chapter opens the book by providing an introduction to ageing and mental health in a global context. It offers an eclectic snapshot of population ageing and mental health issues that affect older people. The chapter briefly discusses the scope, causes, and consequences of population ageing, followed by a discussion on mental health in later life. The chapter highlights the diversity of mental health services for older people in socially, culturally, and geographically different settings. The conclusion of this chapter will provide the structure of the book.

Keywords: population ageing, mental disorder, policy, aged-care, diversity

GLOBAL AGEING AS A REALITY

Populations are rapidly ageing worldwide. Older people increasingly comprise a larger share of the world's total population with a rapid rise in the median age being seen in most societies. While ageing itself is not new to humanity, population ageing is an uncommon phenomenon in human history (World Health Organization [WHO], 2015). It is not just the total world population that is ageing, but the older population itself is growing older (Global

[*] Corresponding author: Hong-Jae Park, The University of Auckland. Email: hj.park@auckland.ac.nz.

Action on Aging, 2001). This unprecedented phenomenon is now a common feature in most nations, cultures and regions, and the trend is expected to continue in coming decades. Consequently, population ageing is set to dominate the social context for the twenty-first century with major social, political, cultural and economic implications (United Nations [UN], 2013).

The following statistics, obtained from the United Nations World Populations Ageing report (2013), give a current snapshot of the world's population ageing landscape. The global share of people aged 60 and over has grown from 9.2% in 1990 to 11.7% in 2013, and is estimated to hit 21.1% by 2050. This translates to more than double the growth of the 841 million people in this age group in 2013 to over 2 billion people by 2050. Consequently, by 2047, the number of older people is projected to be higher than the number of children. As there are more older persons living in low-income countries, and numbers there are growing faster than those of high-income nations, 8 out of 10 of the world's older population will be from less developed regions. Gender differences also feature prominently in population ageing: the majority of older persons are women and their predominance tends to increase with age. At the same time, the proportion of older persons aged 80 years and over (the cohort generally known as "oldest old"), was reported to be at 14% in 2013 and is expected to hit 19% in 2050. If this projection proves correct, this would translate to more than 392 million persons aged 80 years and over by 2050, which is more than three times the present figure.

It is commonly understood that the phenomenon of population ageing stems mainly from the combined effect of fertility declines and longevity increases throughout the world (WHO, 2015). Significantly, a declining fertility rate is the main factor driving population ageing. Fertility has, over a period of time, fallen in most regions of the world, and global fertility rates are projected to continue declining in coming decades. A United Nations' report (2013) shows that the world's total fertility rate has declined by about half, dropping from 5.0 children per woman in the period 1950 – 1955 to 2.5 children per woman in 2010 – 2015. The general trend of individuals leading healthier (and therefore longer) lives is an important contributing factor in the population ageing phenomenon. An increase in life expectancy results in significantly higher proportions of older persons in the total world population. For the high-income nations, population ageing began much earlier than the rest due mainly to more advanced health care systems (UN, 2013). For the period 2010 – 2015, life expectancy is estimated to be at an average 78 years and 68 years in the more and less developed regions, respectively. This increase in life expectancy is projected to continue in coming decades for most regions. By the 2045 – 2050 period, life expectancy for the more developed regions is estimated to average 83 years and 75 years for the less developed regions; this gap is expected to continue to narrow in the following decades (UN, 2013). Furthermore, the ageing 'baby-boomer' cohort (the large cohort born between 1946 and 1964) is an additional factor that escalates this demographic transition in many nations.

Although population ageing is perceived as a global phenomenon, its scope, causes and consequences are not universal. Rather, every country has a unique feature of population ageing, and accordingly, its implications vary on multiple levels. Some countries may have their population growing older rapidly due to the increase in life expectancy and low fertility rates, while populations in other regions remain relatively young due to an influx of migrants and refugees. In some regions, the focus on population ageing might be more on its impact as a whole, while in other regions the concern is more on individuals' ageing experiences. People's attitudes toward population ageing also differ from country to country. For example, a cross-national survey shows that public perceptions about whether the growing number of older people is a social problem vary dramatically from a region to another (Pew Research Center, 2014).

Population ageing itself can be either negative or positive. The consequences of population ageing will depend on how well each society is prepared for these demographic changes. Arguably, ageing societies can be more caring and age-friendly than previously as more seniors contribute to society via family membership, as volunteers, and as active participants in the workforce. In many cultures, older people offer their adult children assistance with babysitting, with some even playing active roles in their grandchildren's school life through attendance at school events. Grandparenting is an increasingly common practice in these societies, with the role of grandparents being acknowledged as a critical structure for supporting the next generation. On the political front, the significance of 'grey power' (the collective power of senior citizens in politics and other social activities) cannot be underestimated as older people have been known to be more active and vote in higher percentages than any other age groups in many nations. However, it is also clear that population ageing results in a range of issues and challenges in many societies, particularly in relation to the care and living arrangements of older people. A common assumption is that, with the rapid growth of population ageing, the number of older people needing health and social care will increase. Especially important is that one of the most immediate consequences of population ageing will be an increase in the number of older people with disabilities and, as a direct result of this, pressures on family support and government finances continue to grow in relation to acute health-care and long-term-care services.

In addition to the increased median age of populations, ageing is also an individual experience. Individual ageing processes will vary significantly from one to another due to differences in health, socio-economic status and historical socialisation backgrounds. Culture plays a significant role in creating different levels of resilience and life outlooks in individuals and families. What is crucial for all to recognise is that each and every human being is, or will potentially become, a member of an ageing society, and that population ageing needs to be considered from a far wider perspective than just ensuring the well-being of the growing number of older people. The development of a sustainable infrastructure in an enabling environment can facilitate the advancement of older people's health, well-being and active participation in society regardless of age factors. Advancements in science and technology are a boon and, innovatively accessed, can benefit initiatives in the management of population ageing.

Mental Health in Late Life

In late adulthood, health is an increasingly crucial issue that affects a person's quality of life, well-being and resilience. As ageing is often associated with a higher prevalence of certain health conditions, healthy ageing becomes a major challenge at different levels and in different settings. Recently, the World Health Organization defined the concept of healthy ageing as "the process of developing and maintaining the functional ability that enables well-being in older age" (WHO, 2015, p. 21). This definition focuses on the older person's functional ability with an equal emphasis on physical and mental health, rather than simply attaching a disease label to the individual. Mental health, like physical health, is essential to the older person's functional ability and happiness. Although perspectives on mental health vary regionally, the World Health Organization's definition is used widely:

> Mental health is not just the absence of mental disorder. It is defined as a state of well-being in which every individual realizes his or her own potential, can cope with the normal stresses of life, can work productively and fruitfully, and is able to make a contribution to her and his community. (WHO, 2014, para 1)

In this sense, most older people have good levels of mental health, coping with stressful life events and other adversities, and strengthening adaptation and resilience throughout their ageing process. Older adults with good mental health are also capable of contributing to their families, communities and the wider society. However, it is crucial to recognise that a considerable proportion of older adults, like people at any stage in the lifespan, are at risk of facing mental health issues. One established theory indicates that the more people age, the more they might develop mental health needs (UN, 2013; WHO, 2014). This theory posits that older people are more likely to be susceptible to certain types of disease, and experience such events as the onset of a physical or mental disability.

The mental health and well-being of older people are influenced, not only by their personal characteristics, but also by the social environments surrounding them within their life-span development context. Multiple biological, psychological and social factors determine levels of mental health in late life, as at any point of time. Culture also influences older people's beliefs in, and perceptions of, mental illness, and their symptomatic expression in certain ways. Especially in old age, people generally begin to reflect more about matters of life and death than at any other life-span stages, and this can affect both their spiritual well-being and mental health. Therefore, it is generally accepted that mental health is inextricably intertwined with physical, emotional, social, cultural, and spiritual health and well-being in later years.

Just as for other age groups, genetic influences and medical conditions can increase the likelihood of mental health issues for older people. Later adulthood is a life period where every individual comes to experience a decline in biological functions and ability to adjust. While some people can sustain good physical health despite their old age, it is inevitable that they will eventually encounter functional declines at a certain stage of late life. As well as the typical life stressors common to all people, many older adults lose their ability to live independently because of limited mobility, chronic pain, frailty, or other physical problems, and might require certain forms of short- or long-term care. Importantly, a person's physical health has an impact on their mental health – and vice versa. For example, older adults with physical health conditions such as heart disease have higher rates of depression than those who are medically well. Conversely, untreated depression in an older person with heart disease can negatively affect the outcome of the disease process (Herbst, Pietrzak, Wagner, White and Petry, 2007).

As people age, their social networks change both in size and quality. Ageing also often creates the need for individuals to make lifestyle changes for a variety of reasons. These changes can have various impacts on the mental health and well-being of older people. In family relations, older people are more likely than ever before to have children or relatives who live in a different location than themselves because of work or other commitments. This results in both parties having limited physical contact and care as personal priorities and circumstances are likely to change. While the role of peers and friends is important in old age, such social networks are also likely to shrink as people age (Charles and Carstensen, 2010). Consequently, the social and emotional life of older people can be affected by the decrease in their roles and social networks. Because people in late life generally have more friends and family members who are dying or terminally ill, bereavement, loss, and grief can be more frequent experiences. This again creates another barrier to meaningful and supportive social networks for older people. Thus, according to Cornwell and Waite (2009), older adults who are socially disconnected have been found to have worse mental health outcomes.

At a more macro level, social environments play an important role in determining the older person's mental capacity and emotional well-being during the ageing process. A significant proportion of older people experience a type of inequality, discrimination, and isolation within social and cultural contexts, and this can contribute to, or deepen and exacerbate, poor mental health and a lack of well-being in later adulthood (Kolb, 2014). Studies have consistently shown that some types of mental health problems are more likely to be prevalent in certain groups of people, such as elderly women in widowhood, seniors in financial instability, and older people in isolation (see, for example, Lai and Surood, 2008). Ageism, referred to as stigma or negative attitudes toward older people, can also have an impact on older adults' mental health and their help-seeking attitudes. All of these factors can contribute to isolation, loss of independence, loneliness and psychological distress, and, thus, have significant impacts on the mental health and well-being of older people across the world.

A range of mental health problems, including neurological disorders, mood disorders and substance-abuse problems, affect the well-being and quality of life of people in later adulthood. These may include dementia, schizophrenia, bipolar disorders, anxiety and depression, post-traumatic stress, and the effects of alcohol or drug misuse (Neno, Aveyard and Heath, 2007). The number of older adults living with mental health problems is growing and approximately 15% of adults aged 60 and over suffer from a mental disorder (WHO, 2014). It is also estimated that approximately 6.6% of the total disability of older adults is attributed to neuropsychiatric disorders. Specifically, more than 47 million people (mostly older adults) around the world suffered from dementia in 2015, and the number of people affected will increase to more than 75 million by 2030 (WHO, 2015). Depression also tends to affect more than 2% of older people living in the community and about 10% of elderly residents in long-term care settings (WHO, 2015). Although generalisation of these figures may be contestable, it is also important to recognise that significant numbers of older adults suffer from mental illnesses for a range of differing reasons in various social and cultural contexts.

Mental Health Policies and Services for Older People

While mental health in late life is a very individual experience, it also constitutes a significant social issue related to stigma, isolation and inequality in service provision and resource allocation. How a society, as a whole, responds to mental health problems can influence the scope and quality of services that older people receive for their illness recovery and quality of life. Comprehensive public-health action and social support systems are required to meet the needs of older people with mental illness. In response, there are a range of legislative acts, social policies and programmes, and practice in health and social services for those people and their families. Public responses need to be complemented by informal care and support for older people with mental health problems in the community. Families, relatives, and neighbours are important sources of care and support for those older people. It is critical that all of these formal and informal responses operate to promote the most effective prevention, treatment, and intervention practices at individual, family, community and societal levels.

Cross-cultural variations in mental health models for older people are significant in the global context where a wide range of cultures are in existence. Cultural values and attitudes towards mental health play an important role in developing health and social policies, and in delivering services and practice for older people from different backgrounds. Social responses to mental health in older people require the development of an enabling socio-cultural environment that facilitates better indicators of an older person's mental health and well-being in the community. Such an inclusive and supportive environment arguably leads to a culturally appropriate framework that allows older people with mental health problems to cultivate a sense of independence, and, thus, be active citizens in their communities (Cornwell and Waite, 2009).

The issue of mental health in older people remains a relatively underdeveloped area, although a significant number of seniors experience mental health issues for a range of differing reasons. In this vein, it can be argued that mental health services for older people have been 'neglected' and, thus, the needs of older people with mental illness have not been met appropriately in many countries (Barker, 2013). Gaps are apparent between service need and service provision, between research and practice, and between formal support and informal care. An inadequate workforce of trained mental health practitioners and other professionals has been an ongoing issue in many nations. Paraprofessionals (including paid-caregivers) are an acknowledged aspect in the care of older people as many of them face burn-out themselves through the stress of heavy workloads particularly in underfunded residential settings (Ellis, Houser and Coughlin, 2014). While the majority of care and support that older people receive are provided by informal caregivers, including family members and relatives, carer support has not been recognised in relation to associated physical, emotional, social and financial stress and burdens.

Although there are major gaps, it is also true that a range of services and initiatives have been developed and implemented to help those older people affected by mental health issues around the world. Legislation, policies and programmes regarding mental health services vary from one nation to another, as well as social and health care systems differing significantly in volume and depth across borders and regions. Cultural differences in mental health and their implications for services are well recognised in some countries, while universal approaches to services are prevalent in others. Diversity in mental health services is significant and has been constantly evolving as more knowledge has accumulated and the practice repertoire has grown in this field.

The purpose of this book is to explore the issues and perspectives associated with mental health in older people around the world. The book will provide an outline of the prevalence, nature and treatment of mental health disorders in the cultural, social, political, and economic contexts that shape selected countries' understanding of and response to these issues. A range of policies and mental health services for older adults with mental illness in individual countries are described. Ultimately, the book will help researchers, policy makers, service providers and students develop their knowledge of the issues, challenges and policies associated with ageing and mental health throughout the world.

THE STRUCTURE OF THE BOOK

This book is one of the first attempts to explore the issues related to mental health and ageing not only in the countries that have been well researched (e.g., the USA), but also the countries where people know little about mental health services for older adults (e.g., Uganda). Apart from this feature, the book provides the same structure for individual chapters. Such a structure offers convenience to readers to compare the cultural context of ageing, prevalence of mental disorders among older adults, mental health services for older people, informal caregiving, policy related to mental health of older people and service and policy gaps, across the countries.

Utilising the Human Development Index in the Human Development Report 2014 (United Nations Development Programme, 2014), the book is structured into three sections. Part I includes eight chapters which discuss mental health and ageing issues, policies and services in high human development countries or regions. Part II presents discussions of mental health in old age in two high- and medium-human-development countries: China and India. Part III focuses on mental health and ageing in Uganda, a low-human-development country.

Chapter 1 provides an introduction to ageing and mental health in a global context by providing a snapshot of population ageing and mental health issues affecting older people. The chapter briefly discusses issues related to the scope, causes and consequences of population ageing, followed by discussion on mental health in late life. Then the chapter draws attention to diversity in mental health services for older people in socially, culturally and geographically different settings.

Next, Chapter 2 discusses the cultural context of ageing in Australia; the prevalence of mental illness among the aged population in that country; services and policies employed to attend to elderly mental health; and the practice of caregiving. The chapter points out that mental illness is prominent among the older population in Australia as the prevalence of mental health issues such as dementia and suicide increase with age. The Australian Government manages most of its age-related policy under the Aged Care Act 1997, and the National Mental Health Strategy Plan. These initiatives stimulate provisions such as Extended at Home Dementia Packages, the National Respite for Carers Program, and the Disability Pension.

A comprehensive picture depicting an increasing awareness of older people's mental health is presented in Chapter 3. It provides an overview of mental health in old age within the context of Switzerland. Without claiming to be exhaustive, it presents information about relevant elements such as Swiss cultural specificities, the prevalence of some important mental disorders affecting the elderly, the services available, the role of caregiving, and some recent policy developments.

In Chapter 4, the prevalence of mental health disorders among older Americans is described as are the context and culture that shape policies about, and service provision for, older adults with mental health disorders. The chapter emphasises that the growth of the older population has spurred heightened awareness of the need to enhance health care provision and ensure the solvency of health care funding for all Americans, especially older adults. The chapter also provides a number of recommendations to enhance the mental health and well-being of the growing population of older Americans.

Chapter 5 provides an outline of mental health and older adults in the New Zealand context. The chapter highlights the cultural initiatives, legislative acts and current programmes in mental health for older people. It discusses the challenges around care for older people with mental health issues. The chapter asserts that new approaches to economic planning are urgently needed, including health care and welfare support, retirement policies, innovative living space arrangements and inter-generational relations alongside the promotion of constructive views on ageing.

The socio-cultural context that shapes Hong Kong's service orientation of mental illness for older adults is examined in Chapter 6. This chapter also reviews mental health services for older adults and caregivers. Through highlighting the challenges related to service development and population ageing as well as the recent initiatives of the Hong Kong Government, the chapter highlights possible directions in translational research. These directions include developing accessible intervention models and advocating strength-based models to empower active older adults in developing sustainable models of care.

The next chapter, Chapter 7, provides an overview of older Koreans' mental health issues by examining multiple aspects: the cultural and contextual aspects, epidemiology of mental disorders in older adults, mental health-related social services and policies, and caregiving issues. Compared to the past practice of aged care where caregiving of older adults was provided mainly by family members, the chapter highlights the new orientation that the Korean government has developed in policies and services to help older citizens and their families. These policies and services include provisions such as National Long-term Care Insurance, Elderly Care Services and the Dementia Management Act.

In Chapter 8, a comprehensive picture of social care for older adults with mental disorders in Japan is provided. It presents the latest available data and information on directions and developments from the mid-1940s to the present day. A highlight of the chapter is a case study indicating how aged care services are applied to an elderly Japanese person with a mental disorder, and why it is necessary to re-evaluate what kinds of care should be provided, and in what circumstances, under the auspices of community care.

The situation of ageing and mental health in Portugal is discussed in Chapter 9. This chapter includes discussions of the prevalence of mental illness among Portuguese; mental health services and caregiving practices among the Portuguese; and the nature of mental health policy in Portugal. The chapter offers insights into the phenomenon that most of Portugal's mental health care is provided generally, and specialised services aimed at older Portuguese are uncommon. Some programmes, such as the National Health Plan, do have specific objectives related to the improvement of older mental health outcomes, but these are not necessarily achieved in practice.

Mental health in old age within the cultural context of filial piety practice and the changes in the one-child policy in China is explored in Chapter 10. The chapter finds that the traditional practice that adult children live with their ageing parents has evolved, resulting in empty-nest households becoming more and more prevalent in China. Along with rapid economic development and urbanisation, the phenomenon of the empty-nest has impacts on the mental health of older Chinese people who may experience loneliness, isolation, and even anxiety and depression.

Chapter 11 looks at the gerontological mental health scenario in India with regard to mental health care policies and services. It deals with old age psychiatry in India; the epidemiology of mental health problems; mental health service needs; delivery of appropriate services within the mental health policy framework; integration of geriatric mental health care into the already existing mental health care service delivery system and training for professionals already working in, or wishing to work in, the field of gerontological mental health in that country.

Mental health systems for older people in Uganda is discussed in Chapter 12. This chapter provides a comprehensive understanding of mental health issues that older people experience within the context of a low-human-development country. The chapter argues that social security benefits are inadequate and, as a result, most elderly people are economically dependent on their children, grandchildren, relatives, and neighbours for survival. Moreover, increasing numbers of older people bear the burden of looking after their grandchildren with limited resources due to death of the parents of the children, mostly from HIV/AIDS.

The last chapter, Chapter 13, offers key conclusions of the book. This chapter further integrates key findings of mental health and ageing from global perspectives. This chapter also discusses how the findings of the book contribute to policy making and to the existing body of knowledge about mental health and ageing.

REFERENCES

Barker, S. (2013). *Caring for older people in nursing*. Los Angeles, CA: Sage.

Charles, S. and Carstensen, L. L. (2010). Social and emotional aging. *Annual Review Psychology, 61*, 383-409.

Cornwell, E. Y. and Waite, L. J. (2009). Social disconnectedness, perceived isolation, and health among older adults. *Journal of Health and Social Behavior, 50*(1), 31-48.

Ellis, D., Houser, A. and Coughlin, J. F. (2014). *An Exploratory Study of Caregiver Stress, Fatigue and Worry in the United States*. MIT AgeLab White Paper No 2014-5. Cambridge, MA: Massachusetts Institute of Technology.

Global Action on Aging. (2001). *Second World Assembly on Ageing: The ageing of the world's population.* Retrieved from http://www.globalaging.org/waa2/documents/theagingoftheworld.htm.

Herbst, S., Pietrzak, R. H., Wagner, J., White, W. B. and Petry, N. M. (2007). Lifetime major depression is associated with coronary heart disease in older adults: Results from the national epidemiologic survey on alcohol and related conditions. *Psychosomatic Medicine, 69*(8), 729-734.

Kolb, P. (2014). *Understanding Aging and Diversity: Theories and Concepts*. New York, NY: Routledge.

Lai, D. and Surood, S. (2008). Predictors of depression in aging South Asian Canadians. *Journal of Cross-Cultural Gerontology, 23*(1), 57-75.

Neno, R., Aveyard, B. and H. B. M. Heath. (2007). *Older people and mental health nursing: A handbook of care*. Malden, MA: Blackwell Publishing.

Pew Research Center. (2014). *Attitudes about Aging: A Global Perspective.* Retrieved from http://www.pewglobal.org/2014/01/30/attitudes-about-aging-a-global-perspective/.

United Nations. (2013). *World population ageing 2013.* Retrieved from http://www.un.org/en/development/desa/population/publications/pdf/ageing/WorldPopulationAgeing2013 54.pdf.

United Nations Development Programme. (2014). Human Development Report 2014. New York, NY: Author.

World Health Organization. (2015) *World Report on Ageing and Health* [Online]. Retrieved from: http://www.who.int/ageing/publications/world-report-2015/en/.

World Health Organization. (2014). *Mental health: A state of well-being.* Retrieved from http://www.who.int/features/factfiles/mental_health/en/.

PART I: VERY HIGH HUMAN DEVELOPMENT COUNTRIES/REGIONS

In: Ageing and Mental Health: Global Perspectives
Editors: Wendy Wen Li, Sherry M. Cummings et al.
ISBN: 978-1-63484-777-3

Chapter 2

AGEING AND MENTAL HEALTH IN AUSTRALIA

Wendy Wen Li* and Kassandra Jackson
James Cook University, Queensland, Australia

ABSTRACT

The health care system in Australia attempts to attend to both physical and mental illnesses. Similar to many developed countries, Australia is increasingly an ageing society, with those over the age of 65 constituting a larger proportion of the population in the past decade than ever before. As a result of this, there is greater pressure on the health care system and on relevant policy to understand and respond to the needs of the elderly. Mental illness is prominent among the older population as the prevalence of mental health issues, such as dementia and suicide, increase with age. The Australian Government manages most of its age related policy under the *Aged Care Act 1997*, and the National Mental Health Strategy Plan. These initiatives stimulate provisions such as Extended at Home Dementia Packages, the National Respite for Carers Program, and the Disability Pension. The present chapter discusses the cultural context of ageing in Australia; the prevalence of mental illness among the aged population in Australia; services and policies employed to attend to elderly mental health; and the practice of caregiving.

Keywords: dementia, depression, anxiety, Indigenous[1] mental health, caregiving, policy

INTRODUCTION

Australia is experiencing a shift in the average age of its population. The growth of this population is largely related to the increased birth rate following the Second World War, commonly referred to as the 'baby boom era' (Australian Bureau of Statistics [ABS], 2004). Improved health care and aged care policy also contribute to higher life expectancy, resulting

* Corresponding author: Wendy Li, James Cook University. Email: wendy.li@jcu.edu.au.

[1] In Australia, Indigenous is a short generic reference covering all Aboriginal and Torres Strait Islander peoples. The word 'Indigenous' is always capitalised when it refers to the original inhabitants of Australia.

in more time as a part of the over 65 age group. Furthermore, the country's fertility rate has not been at replacement level since 1976, and in 2013 was at 1.88 babies per woman (ABS, 2012a). The fertility rate is considered at replacement level when each woman produces enough children to replace herself and her partner. This ageing population means that there are a greater number of older people who may experience mental illness. While most older adults have good mental health, many are at risk of developing mental disorders, neurological disorders, or substance use problems as well as physical illness or disability. Australian research into ageing and mental health is concentrated largely on dementia, depression, and anxiety, and for the most part fails to address other mental health issues. For the Indigenous population, information is especially limited due to lack of research in the area as well as the difficulty involved with applying Western measurements to the Indigenous population.

The present chapter seeks to first discuss the ageing population in Australia and public understandings of ageing. It will then investigate the prevalence of mental illness among older persons for the mainstream population as well as for Indigenous Australians. The available and most commonly sought mental health services as well as general caregiving practices will then be discussed, followed by the policies which serve older people and those suffering mental illness. Finally, gaps in the present understanding of mental disorders in Australian older adults will be identified, leading to suggestions for future research in this area.

Ageing Population and Public Understandings of Ageing in Australia

Australia's population is projected to grow from 21.5 million to between 36.8 and 48.3 million by 2061 (ABS, 2013a). Over this period there will be significant changes to the age structure of the population. In 2011, there were 3 million people aged 65 years and over. This age group is projected to grow to between 9 million and 11.1 million in 2061 (ABS, 2013a). In 2013, the group aged over 75 constituted 6.4% of the population, and by 2060, is expected to constitute 14.4% of the population (Productivity Commission, 2013). Of the Australian population in 2011, approximately 3% (or 669,881) were Indigenous, with around 13% aged over 50 (ABS, 2013b). The average life expectancy among Indigenous Australians in 2012 was somewhat lower than the general population, at 69.1 years for males and 73.7 years for females (ABS, 2013c), compared to 79.9 years for males and 84.3 years for females in the general population (ABS, 2012b). Therefore, Indigenous Australians are considered elderly once they reach 50 years rather than 65. The proportion of those Indigenous Australians aged over 50 is also expected to increase as the general population ages.

Australia consists of five States: New South Wales (NSW), Queensland (QLD), South Australia (SA), Western Australia (WA), and Tasmania; and two Territories: the Northern Territory (NT) and the Australian Capital Territory (ACT). The largest proportion of older people reside in Tasmania (16%) and SA (16%), followed by NSW (14%), Victoria (14%), QLD (13%), WA (12%), the ACT (10%), and finally, the NT (6%). The higher ageing population in Tasmania is attributed to younger adults moving to the mainland from Tasmania due to economic considerations (ABS, 2013c). The lower ageing population in the NT is attributed to the higher Indigenous population whose age profile is younger than the general population, as well as to Darwin (the capital city of the NT) having a higher population of working age individuals.

While the number of Australians aged over 65 years is growing, ageism, the discrimination against older people based on their age, is still common in Australian society. In a study conducted by the Australian Human Rights Commission (AHRC, 2013), participants were asked about their experiences of ageism. For those aged 55-64 years, 35% reported experiencing some form of age-related discrimination, and of those aged 65 or over, this increased to 43%. Most commonly, survey respondents reported being turned down for a position due to their age. They also reported a feeling of invisibility, expressing that they had been ignored in customer service situations and believing that service people did not value time spent on an older person.

Some stereotypes associated with ageing are also endorsed by Australians. In the aforementioned study, participants from a number of age groups were asked about their attitudes towards ageing. Around 44% of Australians felt sorry for older people as they were more likely to suffer complicated health problems, and more than half (51%) of Australians believed that older people were more forgetful. These negative stereotypes can lead to negative behaviors, which can in turn affect the experiences of older individuals. For example, in this study, 20% of Australians reported avoiding discussing technology with older individuals because they believed it would take too much effort (AHRC, 2013).

While ageism and age stereotypes can arise in a variety of ways, the media is in a particularly powerful position to influence perceptions of older people (Hall, 2005). Generally, studies have suggested that older adults are portrayed in positive ways, although less positive than other age groups (Miller, Leyell and Mazachek, 2004). Contrastingly, research has also indicated that older characters in the popular media, such as television, are stereotyped by being presented as ridiculous, cynical, bitter, stubborn, demented, unhealthy, lonely, frail, or as victims (AHRC, 2013; Hall, 2005). Older characters, especially older female characters, were underrepresented in the media compared to census figures. In 2012, although 14.2% of Australia's population was over 65, only 4.7% of those in advertising were of a similar age. Additionally, people over the age of 65 were referred to in only 6.6% of editorial media content (AHRC, 2013). Research has also demonstrated that older characters tend to be present in commercials where health products, food, drinks, services, household products, superannuation, funeral plans, and insurance are promoted (AHRC, 2013; Hall, 2005).

The negative impacts of ageism on the community, older persons and society as a whole are considerable in terms of their economic, social and psychological costs. (AHRC, 2010; Bryant, Bei, Gilson, Komiti and Jackson, 2012). For instance, negative stereotypes and attitudes can influence the mental and physical health of older individuals. Research has shown that older Australians who have a positive attitude towards ageing are more likely to report positive mental and physical health and those with more negative attitudes towards ageing experience more mental and physical illnesses (AHRC, 2013). Moreover, some aspects of stereotypes (e.g., forgetfulness, frailty, vulnerability) may encourage older people to believe that symptoms of mental disorders (e.g., cognitive impairment, depression) are a normal part of ageing. This may discourage them from seeking assistance for mental health issues.

THE PREVALENCE OF MENTAL DISORDERS IN OLDER AUSTRALIANS

Mental disorders affect a significant proportion of older Australians. Often, a mental disorder presents co-morbidly with another mental or physical illness. Due to the physical decline associated with ageing, and the close relationship between dementia, depression, and anxiety, older people are correspondingly more likely to experience mental health problems. Females are more likely than males to report suffering a mental illness, reflecting rates in the general population (ABS, 2013d).

Depression and Anxiety

Due to differences in methodology (e.g., definitions of depression and anxiety, sampling strategies and sample sizes) and measures of depression and anxiety (Li and Miller, 2014), the prevalence of depression and anxiety among older people in literature is inconsistent. Methodological issues aside, the literature generally indicates that depression and anxiety are major mental disorders among older people. It is estimated that around 10% of older Australians experience anxiety and 10-15% experience depression (National Ageing Research Institute [NARI], 2009). Older individuals who receive a high level of home support are nearly twice as likely to develop depression compared to the general population, and it is believed that up to 25% of residents in aged care facilities may be suffering from depression and anxiety. For older people, the more common triggers of anxiety and depression include physical illness and personal loss (Beyondblue, 2013).

The prevalence of depression in the older Indigenous population is difficult to ascertain. In 2014, one study aimed to validate a culturally appropriate scale which assesses depressive disorders in the Kimberley in northern WA. With a sample of 250 participants from an Indigenous background between the ages of 46 and 89, results suggested that depression was present in 7.7% of cases, and was higher for women (10.4%) than men (4.0%) (Alemida et al., 2014). Estimates of depression rates may be influenced by Western methods of measuring, defining, and treating depression. For the Indigenous population, depression may be related to concepts that are non-Western such as loss of land, and so to accurately investigate depression prevalence there must be a culturally relevant assessment. Furthermore, the expression of depression may be different in the Indigenous population, presenting as a weakened spirit or anger, whereas in the mainstream population that might not be the case (Dudgeon, Milroy and Walker, 2014). Therefore, the lack of research into how depression presents among older Indigenous Australians, as well as its prevalence, represents a significant gap in understanding. Investigating this area could improve the outcomes of older Indigenous Australians who are suffering from depression.

Suicide

The highest suicide rates in Australia are observed among older people. In 2012, the highest suicide rate for females was in the 80-84 age group (9.5 suicides per 100,000) and the over 85 age group for males (37.6 suicides per 100,000) (ABS, 2012d). In some cases, suicide has been linked to living alone, hopelessness, and a history of past suicide attempts. Research has suggested that in Australia, those over 60 who commit suicide may be less likely to present with a psychiatric diagnosis compared to other age groups. This suggests that while psychological health is important for older individuals, in considering suicide prevention, it is also necessary to attend to other factors such as the environment, general health, and social life (De Leo, 2013).

Recently, there has been a focus on high suicide rates among the Indigenous population; however, these higher rates are present mainly in the younger population. Older Indigenous people have suicide rates similar to, or slightly lower than, the general population across both genders (ABS, 2010b). Nevertheless, this has increased somewhat from the preceding 15 years (De Leo, Sveticic and Milner, 2011).

Dementia

In Australia, there are over 332,000 individuals living with dementia (Alzheimer's Australia, 2009). It is cited as the leading cause of disability for those aged over 65 years, with over 1,700 new cases diagnosed each week (AIHW, 2012a). It has been reported that 53% of those in aged care suffer from dementia, and a further 26.3% suffer a mental illness other than dementia. Considering that in 2011 there were approximately 169,000 people living in aged care, this constitutes a significant number of individuals (AIHW, 2011a, 2012b). The prevalence of dementia increases with age. In 2008, it was estimated that fewer than 2% of Australians aged between 65 and 74 suffered from dementia, but that nearly 9% of those aged between 75 and 84 suffered dementia (AIHW, 2012a). Among those aged 85 and over, it was estimated that around one in five individuals had dementia. In general, males had lower rates of Alzheimer's disease than females, and this disparity increased with age (AIHW, 2010). While cases of dementia can occur with ageing, it may also occur as a result of alcohol abuse. A study conducted by the Hospital Dementia Services Project using hospital data estimated that in 2006-7 there were around 3500 older people suffering from alcohol related dementia (ARD) across Australia (Draper, 2013).

Although dementia is listed as the most common cause of burden of disease in the older population, it can be managed. Some methods of dementia management include medication, improved diet and exercise, routine, and the introduction of a caregiver. Dementia management differs as dementia increases in severity, from mild assistance and small lifestyle changes to a transition into residential care or a hospice. In the period 2010-11, 10.4% of those between 65 and 74 seeing a general practitioner were able to manage their dementia through implementation of methods such as those mentioned previously. For those aged between 75 and 84, the percentage increased to 41.6%, and for the group aged 85 to 94, it decreased slightly to 38.8%. For those aged 95 years and older, only 5.3% of individuals seeing a GP were managing their dementia (Quinn, 2013).

For Indigenous Australians, dementia prevalence also appears to increase with age. Smith et al. (2008) conducted a study including 363 Indigenous Australians over the age of 45 from the Kimberley region in northern WA and found that around 12.4% presented with dementia. From this same population, it was found that for those over the age of 65 years, the prevalence of dementia increased to 27%. It is worth noting that estimates for dementia prevalence were higher for the Indigenous population than for the general population. While dementia appears to be especially prevalent among the Indigenous population, some research has shown that Indigenous people's knowledge regarding Alzheimer's disease and dementia is relatively limited. Among a sample of 174 Indigenous Australians participating in a modified version of the Alzheimer's disease Knowledge Test, it was found that more than one quarter of older Indigenous Australians (26.5%) had no knowledge regarding Alzheimer's Disease, and more than half (51%) had only some knowledge (Garvey, 2011). It is therefore necessary to increase the availability of information surrounding dementia and Alzheimer's disease for Indigenous Australians to improve the outcomes of those who are suffering from these illnesses.

Psychosis

In 2010, approximately 7,341 individuals between 55 and 64 years sought treatment for a psychotic disorder in the preceding 12 months (Department of Health, 2010). The most common form of psychosis is schizophrenia. It has been suggested that approximately one in every 100 Australians will develop schizophrenia (SANE, 2014), although actual research into its prevalence in the older population is limited. Despite the scarcity of prevalence research, there has been some qualitative investigation into the experiences of older women with schizophrenia. In 2003, researchers conducted a series of interviews with six older, female individuals suffering from schizophrenia. They reported that of these participants, most had been living with the disease since before the 1960s, when the primary methods of treatment were electroconvulsive therapy (ECT) and institutionalisation. Consequently, they were not only coping with the illness, but with the aftermath of its presence in their earlier lives. Because of those early struggles, most participants reported that their lives had improved with age as treatment and their understanding of the illness and themselves increased (Pentland, Miscio, Eastabrook and Krupa, 2003). While participants in this study experienced improved symptoms with age, this may not be true for the next generation of ageing women with schizophrenia because their early treatment and management experiences will be vastly different.

For Indigenous Australians, there is relatively little information available on the prevalence of psychotic disorders. Hunter et al. (2012) conducted an investigation at Cape York and the Torres Strait in far north QLD which looked into psychosis prevalence among 60 Indigenous individuals over the age of 40. In this study, 1.51% of individuals experienced some kind of psychotic disorder (Hunter et al., 2012). Hunter et al. (2011) also reported that males were more likely to suffer from psychotic disorders than females, and schizophrenia was the most commonly reported psychotic diagnosis, followed by substance related psychoses. This research also suggested that in this population psychosis is very complex, and social determinants and context are integral to positive outcomes (Hunter et al., 2011). While this cannot be directly generalised to all Indigenous communities, acknowledging the significance of context and social influences on Indigenous mental health is a positive step towards improved treatment.

Substance Abuse

People over the age of 65 are statistically more likely to be using medications than the general population, likely due to their more prevalent use of sleeping medication. According to national survey data, nearly half of those who reported medicating for mental wellbeing also reported using sleeping medication in the past two weeks (ABS, 2006). This regular use of prescription medications is only one example of a gateway to older adult substance abuse, whether intentional or not.

Older people in Australia have the highest rate of prescription drug abuse than any other age group, with 3% of older individuals admitting to having used pain killers or analgesics for non-medical purposes. Furthermore, many older people continue to consume alcohol regardless of their medication, ignorant of the potentially dangerous side effects (Hunter, 2011). Males appear to be at an increased risk of substance abuse than females, which is in line with prevalence for other age groups. Additionally, in aged care services, around 4.4% of residents report misusing opioids or benzodiazepines (BZ). This is especially concerning due to the recommendation that BZ be avoided by older adults, as it is associated with falls, residual sedative effects, overdoses, and reduced memory capacity (Draper, 2013). Additionally, research has suggested that approximately 25% of the aged population is prescribed five or more drugs for various health needs. These may interact with each other, with alcohol, or cause side effects that consumers are not aware of (AIHW, 2007b). In Australia, the highest number of deaths observed as a result of psychoactive substance abuse was in the 75-84 year old population (AIHW, 2010). Whether this is a result of increased psychoactive drug use, or decreased tolerance for such drugs, is not known.

Alcohol use among the elderly is also an ongoing issue among older Australians. The 2010 National Drug Strategy Household Survey found that approximately 4.3% of individuals aged 65-74, as well as 2.4% of those aged over 75 continued to drink alcohol at levels which placed them at high risk of an injury every day or on most days (Draper, 2013). Furthermore, surveys conducted by the AIHW (2007c) showed that around 15% of individuals over 65 consumed alcohol on a daily basis and 8% used tobacco daily. A later survey by the AIHW showed that having a disability did not increase alcohol consumption (AIHW, 2010). This is especially relevant to the older population because they are more likely to be suffering from a disability than the general population, and it is necessary to acknowledge that disability may not be a driving factor in alcohol consumption. Although alcohol consumption among older people is not popularised in the media, a review of the literature and discussion with relevant practitioners suggested that alcohol is the most common form of substance abuse among individuals over 60 (Hunter, 2011).

While the main substance abuse concerns for older Australians are related to prescription medication and alcohol abuse, as the baby boomers enter the category of 65 years and over, there is some concern that they will bring with them illicit substances and tobacco from their youth. This could potentially create new problems for service providers and policy makers, as this new generation may have different service needs. Coupled with the ageing population, the presence of new and diverse needs among the older population is set to put significant pressure on the aged care and health systems (Hunter, 2011).

Alcohol use is also a concern among older Indigenous Australians. In 2010, the AIHW conducted a review of data compiled from national surveys which investigated alcohol consumption among the Indigenous population. This review reported that approximately 22%

of males between the ages of 45 and 54, and 13% of males over 55 years consumed alcohol to a high-risk level in the 12 months preceding the survey. For females the percentages are lower, at around 14% for those between 45 and 54 years, and 6% for those over 55. Approximately 6 individuals per 1,000 in the over 55 Indigenous population were hospitalised principally due to alcohol use (AIHW, 2011b). According to the 2008 National Aboriginal and Torres Strait Islander Social Survey, 10% of Indigenous individuals over the age of 55 partook in chronic risky or high risk alcohol consumption. This was the lowest percentage among Indigenous Australians, but was still significantly higher than the general population (ABS, 2010). This suggests that older Indigenous Australians are more likely than their mainstream counterparts to be consuming alcohol at a high-risk level.

Mental Health Services for Older Australians

In order to support the ageing population, Australia provides a number of health care services for older Australians suffering from mental illness. While in some cases they are not aimed specifically at mental health, mental illness is often included as a contingency on which one can be eligible for assistance. The main services available aimed directly at elderly mental health are related to dementia, for which there is significant information and support.

A 2007 study by the ABS (2009) reported that 37.3% of those between 55 and 85 years used a service for mental health problems. Of these, 28.9% of individuals reported seeing a general practitioner and 8.7% reported seeing a psychologist. Among the Australian population, this age group was the most likely to see a general practitioner and the least likely to see a psychologist (ABS, 2009). This may be due to the type of mental illnesses suffered by those between 55 and 85 years being more appropriately seen to by a general practitioner, or how general practitioners are perceived compared to psychologists.

As the population ages, it is expected that the required geriatric work force will grow. In 2012, there were only 397 practicing geriatric medicine specialists in Australia and there are ongoing difficulties filling positions in this area. Often those who specialise in geriatric medicine are older themselves, meaning a shorter presence in the workforce. It is also difficult to attract geriatric specialists away from capital cities. It is predicted that by 2025 there will be around 784 geriatric medicine specialists in Australia, with no current plans to attract more individuals to this workforce (Health Workforce Australia, 2012). The number of nurses employed in aged care in 2011 was 40,433, a much higher number than in any other specialisation. This population also had the highest number of enrolled nurses (41.5% of all enrolled nurses), meaning that of those employed in aged care, a large number were enrolled nurses as opposed to registered nurses. Registered nurses have completed a three to three and a half year Bachelor of Science (Nursing) or Bachelor of Nursing at university. Enrolled nurses have completed 12-18 months of full time study for a Diploma of Enrolled Nursing and always work under the supervision of a registered nurse (Government of Western Australia, 2013). Like geriatric medicine, nurses in aged care are also more likely to be older than those in other nursing fields (AIHW, 2011c). Since 2003, the number of both enrolled and registered nurses employed in aged care has fallen. This may be because workers in that area can expect a lower remuneration rate than those in similar roles elsewhere, and an increasing trend toward employing less skilled staff in residential settings (Health Workforce

Australia, 2013). The number of nurses employed in mental health in 2011 was 17,738 (AIHW, 2011c). Those working in mental health do not necessarily work with older individuals, and no information was available regarding an approximate number of psychogeriatric nurses specifically. However, it has been suggested that there has been a decline in psychogeriatric nursing positions, with mental health nurses filling these roles instead (Jeon, n.d.).

In Australia, responsibility for maintaining mental health is shared by State and Federal governments. The Federal Government has approached mental health through the *National Mental Health Strategy* over the previous three decades (AIHW, 2014). This has led to the development of a number of *National Mental Health Plans*, as well as the *Roadmap for National Mental Health Reform 2012-2022*, the purpose of which is to provide a pathway towards an Australian society that values good mental health and wellbeing. It was developed together by Commonwealth, State, and Territory governments and will assist in deciding where to direct investments, how to design policy, and to understand the path that leads to achieving good mental health and wellbeing nationwide. The roadmap recognises the importance of each level of government in the delivery of mental health care and support services. The state governments are primarily responsible for hospital based, specialised, and community based mental health services aimed at those with severe or persistent mental illness. The Commonwealth Government's principal role is to support primary care. Such services are delivered through Medicare as well as through the funding of non Government organisations and the Pharmaceutical Benefits Scheme (PBS).

In Australia, the basis of the health care system is Medicare, which covers many health care costs including hospital treatment and seeing a doctor within a hospital. Medicare also subsidises visits to doctors outside of hospitals including specialists. Furthermore, it sits alongside the PBS which subsidises some medications. All Australian citizens and most permanent residents are eligible for Medicare (Department of Human Services, 2015). As of 2012-13, those over the age of 65 were less likely to be using any kind of Medicare subsidised mental health services including psychiatrists, general practitioners, and psychologists than any other adult group. These statistics may reflect the overall reduced likelihood of those over 65 seeking assistance for mental health, and suggests that they are also less likely to take advantage of Medicare subsidised services (AIHW, 2013a).

The Australian Government also funds residential aged care, community care, and a number of other aged care support programs. In 2011-12, approximately 10% of individuals over the age of 70 were being provided with permanent residential care; approximately 3.6% of those over 70 were receiving a community care package such as the Community Aged Care Package or the Extended Aged Care at Home Dementia (EACHD) package; 2.1% of those over 70 received residential respite care; and 21,730 people were provided with care under the Transition Care Program. Some individuals received care under more than one of these programs (Department of Health and Ageing [DoHA], 2012). The EACHD package is one of the few aimed specifically at mental health care. It provides high level care to those with dementia in their own homes and is relatively flexible, generally offering assistance with transport, continence, emotional and social support, as well as practical benefits such as home safety modifications (Doyle and Haralambous, 2012). Moreover, those with dementia are eligible for support under the PBS and Repatriated PBS (RPBS). In 2008-09, more than 386,000 prescriptions for four different drugs provided to treat Alzheimer's were subsidised by the PBS and RPBS schemes combined (AIHW, 2010).

Psychogeriatric units (PGUs) also provide support for older individuals with mental illnesses. PGUs are wards within hospitals where care is provided for older individuals experiencing illnesses such as psychosis and mood disorders. They also provide care for patients with challenging behavior resulting from mental illness (Dobrohotoff and Llewellyn-Jones, 2011). Like other countries, Australian PGUs provide a varied experience, even within the same state. In a survey of 200 NSW public hospitals, it was found that 8% of hospitals had beds specifically for the specialist mental health treatment of older persons. On average, each of these hospitals had 15 beds. General hospitals also contained acute aged care beds (average of 39), but they were not specifically for those requiring mental support (Draper, 2010). Furthermore, use of restraint and seclusion are inconsistent across PGUs. In Victoria, five PGUs comparable for environment and staffing reported vastly different usage of restraint and seclusion (O'Connor et al., 2004). Across the PGUs, varying methods of restraint (for example, having the patient sit in a beanbag as opposed to physically restrained) were used, and in two PGUs, seclusion rooms were not used. It has been suggested that seclusion rooms may not be required at all, even for patients with the most challenging behavior. This is just one area in which PGUs in Australia require further investigation.

The Australian Government also provides funding to not-for-profit organisations to work with older Australians with mental illness and their carers. One such group is Alzheimer's Australia. The funding provided aims to assist them in delivering the National Dementia Support Program (NDSP), which provides counseling and support, early intervention programs, and education and training. Furthermore, Alzheimer's Australia provides support specifically for Indigenous Australians, people from culturally and linguistically diverse backgrounds, people from rural and remote areas, and those who are gay, lesbian, bisexual, transgender, or intersex. They also maintain a national dementia hotline (Alzheimer's Australia, n.d.; DoHA, 2012). Beyondblue also provides support for those suffering from both anxiety and depression, and has recently initiated the Professional Education to Aged Care (PEAC) program. This program aims to train and educate carers and professionals about depression and anxiety in older individuals. This is especially helpful as dementia often facilitates depression, and the symptoms of dementia, depression, and anxiety can often appear similar (Beyondblue, 2012).

State governments also provide assistance to older Australians suffering mental illness. While their services vary, they often fund carer assistance programs, dementia support and home help, and provide information to the community (McIntosh and Phillips, 2003). Furthermore, states often provide discounts through Seniors' Cards or transport assistance which may help decrease social isolation and increase independence, which are both significant factors contributing to mental health. For example, the NSW government, in conjunction with the Australian Government, promotes the Home and Community Care Program. The purpose of this program is to help older people stay at home longer by providing activities, transportation, home maintenance or modification, and household chores (NSW Government, 2013). There are also services specifically for Indigenous Australians, including some specialist state government services. For example, the Department of Health in WA provides a Specialist Aboriginal Mental Health Services (SAMHS) which aims to be holistic and culturally appropriate, involving elders and traditional healers in the service process (Government of Western Australia, n.d.). There has also been some research into the determinants of mental health service usage among older Indigenous Australians. In 2011, the NSW Government conducted a report into mental health service use through workshops with older Indigenous Australians, community members, and service providers, as well as an online survey of service providers. It suggested that older Indigenous people are more likely to access services which have received positive reports from other Indigenous people and less likely to use services which have received negative reports. Furthermore, they prefer to access services which build community relationships, are culturally competent, and provide appropriate health promotion materials (NSW Department of Health, 2010).

INFORMAL CAREGIVING FOR OLDER AUSTRALIANS WITH MENTAL DISORDERS

In 2011, around 2.9 million Australians were providing support to a friend or family member suffering from mental illness, a chronic condition, a terminal illness, or who was aged (Healey, 2012). Informal caregiving is most often carried out by women, and it is estimated that informal care accounts for around 75% of care provided to older people and to those with disabilities (Women's Health Victoria, 2008).

Informal caregiving can have a significant impact on the daily life of carers. In Australia, the overall time provided by carers in 2010 was approximately 1.32 billion hours. It was estimated that around 129,900 carers could not maintain employment because of their caring responsibilities, representing a significant loss of income (Access Economics, 2010a). Furthermore, carers themselves sometimes experience detriments to their health and wellbeing. It has been reported that those caring for someone with dementia, especially long term family carers, can have increased general stress, depression, and anxiety. This can lead to physical health impacts and disrupted sleep. To alleviate such stressors, it is important to provide carers with appropriate and flexible support (Access Economics, 2009). The relationship between the caregiver and recipient may also affect the wellbeing of the carer. It has been reported that parents experience more satisfaction and positive affect than spouses when fulfilling the role of carer, and adult children report the least amount of satisfaction. Spouses are more likely to experience depression than parents and children of the care recipient when the recipient has dementia (Savage and Bailey, 2004). Some research has also suggested that caregivers who live with their recipients experience a greater negative effect on well-being (Savage and Bailey, 2004).

Caregiving requirements can influence living arrangements. In 2012, only 8.2% of those over the age of 65 reported living with a child or other relative; however, 38% of those required some kind of assistance, and this percentage increased with age (ABS, 2011). Therefore, those living with a child or relative are more likely to be living with them out of a need for care as they grow older. This may be even more prevalent in Indigenous communities, where research into caregiving in later life in the NT has suggested that older Indigenous people often want their family members to be around them (McGrath, 2008).

While older people can require care, they often fulfill the role of carers themselves. In 2009, 20% of all carers were aged over 65, despite this age group constituting only 13% of the total population, and nearly 80% of those were caring for their partner. Older people acting as carers can experience physical and emotional detriment as a result of their role. In 2009, nearly one quarter (24%) of those caring for another reported feeling frequently worried or depressed (ABS, 2012c). As a result of often being carers themselves, older Australians may benefit from the *National Respite for Carers Program* provided by the Australian Government. This program provides short term care so that carers have the opportunity to take a break from full time caring. Respite care may be provided for a few hours or for weeks depending on the requirements of the carer and the person they care for. It may also take place in the home, or involve moving the person cared for into an aged care facility temporarily. There were 109,210 carers in 2011-12 who received assistance under this program (DoHA, 2012).

The future supply of informal care is likely to be affected by the ageing population and changing social constructs. Presently, females are more likely to be carers than males, so increasing female workforce participation somewhat reduces the pool of potential carers. Additionally, smaller family sizes and increased divorce rates further serve to limit the pool of potential carers (Access Economics, 2010b). Generational differences may also affect informal caregiving, with individuals from generations X and Y (born between the late 1960s and early 2000s) being less prepared than Baby Boomers to provide primary care. This is suspected to be because of the known detriments to health and well being, and the potentially more individualistic nature of the younger generations (Access Economics, 2009). These factors combined may place further strain on the aged care system as the population ages.

MENTAL HEALTH POLICIES RELATED TO OLDER PEOPLE

In Australia, most government initiated aged care services exist under the *Aged Care Act 1997*. The government's description of the Act itself is relatively limited in terms of any specific discussion on mental health. However, it does provide stimulation for some of the aforementioned government policies and programs such as the *National Mental Health Strategy, National Respite for Carers Program*, *Community Aged Care Packages*, and *Disability Support Pension*.

The *National Mental Health Strategy* was implemented in 1992 and has been developed, revised, and reaffirmed over time to reflect society and the evolving understanding of mental illness. The Strategy's primary purpose is to promote the overall health of the Australian community; to reduce the impact and presence of mental health disorders; and to ensure that those with a mental illness are able to maintain their rights. It also seeks to develop awareness and understanding throughout the community, so that members are able to more easily recognise and cope with mental illness whether it is experienced by themselves or those around them (Commonwealth of Australia, 2009).

In 2010, the *National Health and Hospital's Network Agreement* (NHHN) was announced to set out the architecture and foundations of the National Health and Hospitals Network. This is an agreement between the Commonwealth of Australia and its States and Territories to improve health outcomes, including for the elderly and mentally ill, and maintain a sustainable health care system (Council of Australian Governments [COAG], 2010). Regarding elderly mental health specifically, some have suggested that the NHHN agreement attends mainly to acute needs. This means that elderly people in the community who suffer mild mental illness are unable to seek help through this service, leading to their condition worsening until they require the acute services offered (Mental Health Council of Australia, 2010).

In 2012, COAG produced a roadmap for the future of mental health in Australia spanning from 2012 until 2022 (Commonwealth of Australia, 2012). It is a health reform plan that promotes a positive ageing experience by supporting independence and lifestyle maintenance of older Australians. Australia's ageing society means that more people leave the workforce than enter it, which presents certain economic challenges as well as increased pressure on health and aged care services. Ensuring that older individuals remain independent and industrious members of the community means that they are able to support society for longer, subsequently reducing these pressures.

In 2013, The Australian Government released a resource sheet detailing *Strategies and practices for promoting the social and emotional wellbeing of Aboriginal and Torres Strait Islander people*. This resource sheet promotes the notion that Indigenous cultures take a holistic view of life and health; therefore cultural, spiritual, and social wellbeing are integral to the health of Indigenous people. It also acknowledges that the impact of colonisation, relocation of people to missions and reserves, and the forced removal of children resulted in the dispossession and dislocation of Aboriginal and Torres Strait Islander people from land and family. This has disrupted cultural beliefs and practices, and has adversely affected the social and emotional wellbeing of Indigenous people (AIHW, 2013b).

Policy and Service Gaps and Recommendations

There are a number of policy and service gaps which are evident upon reviewing the available literature. Improvements in treatment investment, services, and research funding would increase the knowledge available regarding older mental illness. Additionally, there are significant gaps in knowledge surrounding prevalence and appropriate treatment of mental illness among the Indigenous population. Finally, the mental health literacy of the older population and Australians in general appears to be relatively limited, which appears to further exacerbate negative stereotypes and ideas about ageing.

Policy Gaps

While there are a number of policies dedicated to the maintenance of mental health as well as to ageing, their investment in treatment, services, and research is limited. Often the policies provide guidelines as to how the state of mental health or ageing should be handled without necessarily providing the funds to follow through. Furthermore, policies and services to attend to older mental illness are often separate, with each maintaining its own goals and ideals. By instead approaching mental illness for the ageing population holistically, treatment and services may be designed in a way that is more specialised. Services can be tailored specifically for older Australians, when presently they are often aimed just at the ageing or just for people with mental illness.

Mental health policy should also address mental health literacy. Within Australia, mental health literacy receives little attention, despite a review conducted by Jorm (2012) showing that mental health illiteracy can significantly influence help seeking behaviors as well as the reception of diagnoses and treatment. Therefore, by incorporating mental health literacy into policy, society will be more efficient at seeking help, improve preventative measures, feel supported by those around them, and see mental health services as valuable assets meriting support from the public and government.

Indigenous Services and Research

Across the literature, there is very little which addresses the mental health needs and experiences of older Indigenous Australians. While some studies have looked into general or Indigenous mental health, the mental health of those over 50 is only infrequently attended to (Hunter et al., 2012, 2011; Smith et al., 2008). This lack of knowledge in some ways precludes governments and service providers from providing culturally appropriate care. Furthermore, research has illustrated that the symptoms of depression among older Indigenous people may be related to culturally specific concepts. Research into mental illness in far north QLD has provided some insight into the needs and priorities of Indigenous Australians when treating mental illness including the emphasis on a holistic treatment method (Hunter et al., 2011). It would be beneficial to develop similar projects in other areas of Australia to further investigate the needs of this population. This would allow service providers to engage appropriately with Indigenous Australians and create awareness of the specific needs and values that are unique to Indigenous culture.

In addition to independent research, it would be beneficial for the government to take advantage of research it conducts routinely to investigate mental illness in the older Indigenous population. For example, surveys such as the People Living with Psychotic Illness 2010 (Morgan et al. 2011), which is conducted every ten years, could incorporate questions requesting the cultural background of participants, and use that information to inform service development.

Education

While ageing and mental health are both the subject of increasing attention in Australia, stereotypes, mental health illiteracy, limited understanding of mental health, and ignorance continue to permeate the experience of ageing. Stereotypes are perhaps the most pertinent issue experienced by older individuals on a daily basis. Not only does it preclude them from the same respect and attention afforded to other age groups, but it encourages negative self image and feelings of worthlessness (AHRC, 2013). Companies selling products and services are recommended to include older people in their advertising, especially as Australia's older population increases. Furthermore, the media should strive to include stories of achievement and positive experiences associated with older individuals, rather than only negative stories which serve to perpetuate notions of vulnerability and fragility. This could improve the self esteem and self worth of the growing elderly population and assist in dissolving the negative stereotypes surrounding ageing.

According to Jorm (2000, 2012), mental health literacy has been the subject of relatively little research and attention. Jorm et al. (2005) suggested that within Australia, there is evidence that when presented with a case scenario, individuals are typically unable to identify a mental illness. Furthermore, in a study involving 273 referrals to a specialist anxiety treatment clinic, individuals took an average of 6.9 years to recognise that they were experiencing a mood or anxiety disorder, after which it took an average of 8.2 years to seek help (Thompson, Issakidis and Hunt, 2008). Lack of understanding that a mental illness is present is a barrier to help seeking. This implies a need for further mental health education. A number of ways to improve mental health literacy include education on disorder recognition, improvement in service knowledge, and prevention methods (Jorm, 2012).

Considering the high rates of medication, substance abuse, and alcohol use among older Australians, more education regarding the interaction between medications and the body should be made available. It may be that some older people are unaware of the body's reduced ability to process alcohol and other substances into old age; therefore, it is necessary to provide education which illustrates how such substances affect the body differently at different points during life. Furthermore, more education on how different medications interact with alcohol may help reduce the frequency and amount of alcohol consumed by the older population. Increasing education will help reduce the likelihood of older people unknowingly taking multiple medications that could have a negative effect on their physical or mental health. It may also serve to discourage those who are purposefully partaking in substance abuse as they may not understand the real damage they are doing.

Finally, knowledge surrounding Alzheimer's disease and dementia among indigenous Australians is relatively limited. Increasing research in this area would allow service providers to disseminate knowledge and information in a culturally appropriate way. This could improve outcomes for those who suffer from this illness as well as their family members, as they would be able to better manage their dementia as well as plan for the future.

CONCLUSION

The present chapter reviewed the mental health issues experienced by older Australians. An overview of Australia's ageing population was provided and the prevalence of mental health problems for both the mainstream and Indigenous populations were investigated. It is evident that there are higher rates of mental illness such as dementia, as well as higher rates of suicide among the older population. Due to the ageing population, these issues will become more prevalent as time passes, which is reflected in policy and service provision for older adults and the Government's preparation for the future. Improved policy and service attention to the specific needs of the elderly, and an approach which addresses mental illness in older Australians from a holistic and educated standpoint may serve to relieve pressure on future health care and improve outcomes for individuals. Older Indigenous mental health issues are especially under-researched, and investment in this area would inform a culturally respectful and appropriate perspective from which to design services, creating benefits for service providers and clients. Finally, increased mental health education for older individuals would improve mental health literacy and individuals' ability to manage mental illness. Furthermore, altering the way older people are portrayed in the media may serve to discredit many of the negative stereotypes surrounding ageing, improving the day to day lives of older people with mental illnesses.

REFERENCES

Access Economics (2009). *Making choices: Future dementia care: Projections, problems and preferences.* Retrieved from https://fight dementia.org.au/sites/default/files/20090400_ Nat__AE_FullMakingChoices.pdf.

Access Economics (2010a). *The economic value of informal care in 2010.* Retrieved from http://carersaustralia.com.au/storage/Economic-Value-Informal-Care-Oct-2010.pdf.

Access Economics (2010b). *Caring places: Planning for aged care and dementia 2010-2050 Volume 1.* Retrieved from https://www.deloitteaccess economics.com.au/uploads/File/ Alzheimers%20Vol1Final%200710.pdf.

Almeida, O. P., Flicker, L., Fenner, S., Smith, K., Hyde, Z., Atkinson, D., … LoGiudice, D. (2014). The Kimberly assessment of depression of older indigenous Australians: Prevalence of depressive disorders, risk factors and validation of the KICA-dep Scale. *PLoS ONE, 9*(4). Doi: 10.1371/journal.pone.0094983.

Alzheimer's Australia (2009). *Keeping dementia front of mind: Incidence and prevalence 2009-2050.* Retrieved from fightdementia.org.au.

Alzheimer's Australia (n.d.). *Services and programs we provide.* Retrieved from https://fightdementia.org.au/support-and-services/services-and-programs-we-provide.

Australian Bureau of Statistics (2004). *Australian social trends, 2004.* (cat no. 4102.0). Retrieved from http://www.abs.gov.au.

Australian Bureau of Statistics (2006). *Mental health in Australian: A snapshot, 2004-05.* (cat no. 4824.0.55.001. Retrieved from http://www.abs.gov.au.

Australian Bureau of Statistics (2009). *Australian social trends, March 2009.* (cat no. 4102.0). Retrieved from http://www.abs.gov.au.

Australian Bureau of Statistics (2010). *The health and welfare of Australia's Aboriginal and Torres Strait Islander peoples, Oct 2010* (cat no. 4704.0). Retrieved from http://www.abs.gov.au.

Australian Bureau of Statistics (2011). *Reflecting a nation: Stories from the 2011 census, 2012-2013* (cat no. 2071.0). Retrieved from http://www.abs.gov.au.

Australian Bureau of Statistics (2012a). *Births, Australia, 2012.* (cat no. 3301.0). Retrieved from http://www.abs.gov.au.

Australian Bureau of Statistics (2012b). *Deaths, Australia, 2012* (cat no. 4102.0). Retrieved from http://www.abs.gov.au.

Australian Bureau of Statistics (2012c). *Australian social trends, Dec 2012* (cat no. 4102.0). Retrieved from http://www.abs.gov.au.

Australian Bureau of Statistics (2012d). *Causes of death, Australia, 2012* (cat no. 3303.0). Retrieved from http://www.abs.gov.au.

Australian Bureau of Statistics (2013a). *Gender indicators, Australia, Jan 2013* (cat no. 4125.0). Retrieved from http://www.abs.gov.au.

Australian Bureau of Statistics (2013b). *Estimates of Aboriginal and Torres Strait Islander Australians, June 2011* (cat no. 3238.0.55.01). Retrieved from http://www.abs.gov.au.

Australian Bureau of Statistics (2013c). *Migration, Australia, 2011-12 and 2012-13, 2013* (cat no. 3412.0). Retrieved from www.abs.gov.au.

Australian Bureau of Statistics (2013d). *Population by age and sex, regions of Australia, 2013* (cat no. 3235.0). Retrieved from www.abs.gov.au.

Australian Human Rights Commission. (2010). *Age discrimination - exposing the hidden barrier for mature age workers*. Sydney: Author.

Australian Human Rights Commission (2013). *Fact or fiction? Stereotypes of older Australians*. Retrieved from http://www.humanrights.gov.au.

Australian Institute of Health and Welfare (2007a). *Older Australia at a glance (fourth edition)*. Retrieved from www.aihw.gov.au.

Australian Institute of Health and Welfare (2007b). *Older Australians in hospital*. Retrieved from www.aihw.gov.ac.

Australian Institute of Health and Welfare (2007c). *National drug strategy household survey*. Retrieved from www.aihw.gov.au.

Australian Institute of Health and Welfare (2010). *Australia's health 2010*. Retrieved from www.aihw.gov.au.

Australian Institute of Health and Welfare (2011a). *Australia's welfare 2011* (Tenth biennial report). Canberra: Author.

Australian Institute of Health and Welfare (2011b). *Substance use among Aboriginal and Torres Strait Islander people* (cat no. IHW 40). Retrieved from www.aihw.gov.au.

Australian Institute of Health and Welfare (2011c). *Nursing and midwifery workforce 2011*. (cat no. HWL 48). Retrieved from www.aihw.gov.au.

Australian Institute of Health and Welfare (2012a). *Dementia in Australia*. (cat no. AGE 70). Retrieved from www.aihw.gov.au.

Australian Institute of Health and Welfare (2012b). *Residential aged care in Australia 2010-11: A statistical overview*. Retrieved from www.aihw.gov.au.

Australian Institute of Health and Welfare (2013a). *Medicare-subsidised mental health related services*. Retrieved from mhsa.aihw.gov.au.

Australian Institute of Health and Welfare (2013b). *Strategies and practices for promoting the social and emotional wellbeing of Aboriginal and Torres Strait Islander people* [Resource sheet no. 19]. Retrieved from www.aihw.gov.au.

Australian Institute of Health and Welfare (2014). *National mental health policies*. Retrieved from mhsa.aihw.gov.au.

Beyondblue (2012). *Beyondblue to tackle depression and anxiety in aged care sector*. Retrieved from http://www.beyondblue.org.au/media/media-releases/media-releases/beyondblue-to-tackle-depression-and-anxiety-in-aged-care-sector.

Beyondblue (2013). *Anxiety and depression in older people*. Retrieved from http://www.beyondblue.org.au/.

Bryant, C., Bei, B., Gilson, K, Komiti, A. and Jackson, H. (2012). The relationship between attitudes to aging and physical and mental health in older adults. *International Psychogeriatrics, 24*(10), 1674-1683. Retrieved from search.proquest.com.

Commonwealth of Australia (2009). *Fourth national mental health plan*. Retrieved from http://www.health.gov.au/internet/main/publishing.nsf/Content/9A5A0E8BDFC55D3BCA257BF0001C1B1C/$File/plan09v2.pdf.

Council of Australian Governments (2010). *National health and hospitals network agreement*. Retrieved from www.0.health.nsw.gov.au.

De Leo, D., Sveticic, J. and Milner, A. (2011). Suicide in Indigenous People in Queensland, Australia: Trends and Methods, 1994-2007. *Australian and New Zealand Journal of Psychiatry, 45*(7), 532-538. Doi: 10.3109/00048674.2011.570310.

De Leo, D. (2013). Suicides in older adults: A case-control psychological autopsy study in Australia. *Journal of Psychiatric Research, 47*(7), 980-988. Doi: 10.1016/ j.jpsychires.2013.02.009.

Department of Health (2010). *People living with psychotic illnesses 2010*. Retrieved from health.gov.au.

Department of Health and Ageing (2012). *2011-12 Report on the operation of the* Aged Care Act 1997. Retrieved from www.health.gov.au.

Department of Human Services (2015). Medicare services. Retrieved from: www.humanservices.gov.au.

Dobrohotoff, J. T., Llewellyn-Jones, R H. (2011). Psychogeriatric inpatient unit design: a literature review. *International Psychogeriatrics, 23*(2), 174-189. Doi: http://dx.doi. org.elibrary.jcu.edu.au/10.1017/S10416102 10002097.

Doyle, C. and Haralambous, B. (2012). *Culturally and linguistically diverse Australians: Population perspectives and research priorities* [Conference paper]. Retrieved from www.cultural diversity.com.au.

Draper, B. (2011). *The Hospital Dementia Services Project: Dementia services provided in NSW public hospitals, Australia.* Presented at the International Psychogeriatric Association 2010 International Meeting. Retrieved from http://www.aihw.gov.au/ WorkArea/DownloadAsset.aspx?id=10737419323&libID=10737419322.

Draper, B. (2013). *If you can remember the 60s you weren't there... Older people and substance misuse*. Presented at Medicine in Addiction 2013 conference. Retrieved from https://www.ranzcp.org/Files/Conference/MIA2013/MiA-Presentations/1225-1245-Draper.aspx.

Dudgeon, P., Milroy, H. and Walker, R. (eds.) (2014). *Working together: Aboriginal and Torres Strait Islander mental health and wellbeing principles to practice*. Retrieved from aboriginal.telethonkids.org.au.

Garvey, G. (2011). Making sense of dementia: understanding amongst indigenous Australians. *International Journal of Geriatric Psychiatry, 26*(6), 649-656. Doi: 10.1002/gps.2578.

Government of Western Australia (2013). Pathways. Retrieved from www.nursing. health.wa.gov.au.

Government of Western Australia (n.d). Statewide and Tertiary Mental Health Services. Retrieved from www.nmahsmh.health.wa.gov.au.

Hall, J. (2005). Television and positive ageing in Australia. Unpublished PhD thesis, Murdoch University, Perth, Australia. Healey, J. (2012). *Carers: Ageing and Disability*. Retrieved from reader.elib.com.au.

Healey, J. (ed.) (2012). *Carers: Ageing and disability*. Thirroul, Australia: The Spinney Press.

Health Workforce Australia (2012). *Health workforce 2025: Medical Specialties Volume 3*. Retrieved from https://www.hwa.gov.au/sites/uploads/HW2025_V3_FinalReport 20121109.pdf.

Health Workforce Australia (2013). *Australia's health workforce series: Nurses in focus*. Retrieved from https://www.hwa.gov.au/sites/default/files/Nurses-in-Focus-FINAL.pdf.

Hunter, B. (2011). *Older people and alcohol and other drugs*. Retrieved from http://www. druginfo.adf.org.au/attachments/445_PRQ_15_Sep11.pdf.

Hunter, E. M., Gynther, B. D., Anderson, C. J., Onnis, L. L., Groves, A., Nelson, J. (2011). Psychosis and its Correlates in a Remote Indigenous Population. *Australasian Psychiatry, 19*(5), 434-438. Doi: 10.3109/10398562.2011.583068.

Hunter, E. M., Gynther, B. D., Anderson, C. J., Onnis, L. L., Nelson, J. R., Hall, W., ... and Groves, A. R. (2012). Psychosis in Indigenous populations of Cape York and the Torres Strait. *The Medical Journal of Australia, 196*(2), 133-135. Doi: 10.5694/mja11.10118.

Jeon, Y. H. (n.d.). *Psychogeriatric nursing workforce in Australia: An endangered species?* Retrieved from http://www.ipa-online.org/wordpress/about-ipa/about-ipa/ipa-news-and-media/workforce-issues/psychogeriatric-nursing-workforce-in-australia-an-endangered-species/.

Jorm, A. F. (2000). Mental health literacy: Public knowledge and beliefs about mental health disorders. *The British Journal of Psychiatry, 177*, 396-401. Doi: 10.1192/bjp.177.5.396.

Jorm, A. F. (2012). Mental health literacy: Empowering the community to take action for better mental health. *American Psychologist, 67*(3), 231-243. Retrieved from search.proquest.com.elibrary.jcu.edu.au.

Jorm., A. F., Nakane, Y., Christensen, H., Yoshioka, K., Griffiths, K. M. and Wata, Y. (2005). Public beliefs about treatment and outcome of mental disorders: a comparison of Australian and Japan. *BMC Medicine, 3*(12). Doi: 10.1186/1741-7015-3-12.

Li, W. and Miller, D. (2014). Mental health and mental capital: Using positive psychology to inform social work practice with older people. In: A. Francis, V. Pulla, M. Clark, S. E. Mariscal and I. Ponnuswami (eds.). Advancing social work in mental health through strengths-based practice (pp. 120-130). Brisbane, Australia: Primrose Hall Publishing.

McGrath, P. (2008). Family care giving for Aboriginal peoples during end-of-life: Findings from the Northern Territory. *Journal of Rural and Tropical Public Health, 7*, 1-10.

McIntosh, G. and Phillips, J. (2003). *'Caring for the Elderly' – an overview of aged care support and services in Australia*. Retrieved from www.aph.gov.au.

Mental Health Council of Australia (2010). *Mental health council of Australia submission to: The productivity commission inquiry into aged care July 2010.* Retrieved from www.pc.gov.au.

Miller, D., Leyell, T. S. and Mazachek, J. (2004). Stereotypes of the elderly in U.S. television commercials from the 1950s to the 1990s. *International Journal of Aging and Human Development, 58*, 315-340.

Morgan, V. A., Waterreus, A., Jablensky, A., Mackinnon, A., McGrath, J. J., Bush, R. ... and Saw, S. (2011). *People living with psychotic illness 2010.* Retrieved from www.health.gov.au.

National Ageing Research Institute (2009). *Beyondblue depression in older age: a scoping study.* (Final Report). Melbourne: Author.

NSW Department of Health (2010). *Aboriginal older peoples' mental health project report 2010.* Retrieved from www.health.nsw.gov.au.

NSW Government (2013). Help at home. Retrieved from www.adhc.nsw. gov.au.

Pentland, W., Miscio, G., Eastabrook, S. and Krupa, T. (2003). Aging women with schizophrenia. *Psychiatric Rehabilitation Journal, 26*(3), 290-302. Retrieved from search.proquest.com.

Productivity Commission (2013). *An Ageing Australia: Preparing for the Future.* Retrieved from www.pc.gov.au.

Queensland Health (2013). *The road to recovery – a history of mental health services in Queensland 1859-2009.* Retrieved from www.health.qld.gov.au.

Quinn, J. (ed.) (2014). *Dementia*. Retrieved from reader.eblib.com.au.elibrary.jcu.edu.au.

SANE Australia (2014). *Schizophrenia* [Fact Sheet]. Australia: Author.

Smith, K., Flicker, L., Lautenschlager, N. T., Almeida, O. P., Atkinson, D., Dwyer, A. and LoGuidice, D. (2008). High prevalence of dementia and cognitive impairment in Indigenous Australians. *Neurology, 71*(19), 1470-1473. Doi: 10.1212/01.wnl.0000320508.11013.4f.

Thompson, A., Isaakidis, C. and Hunt, C. (2008). Delay to Seek Treatment for Anxiety and Mood Disorders in an Australian Clinical Sample. *Behaviour Change, 25*(2), 71-84. Doi: http://dx.doi.org/10.1375/bech.25.2.71.

Women's Health Victoria (2008). *Women and informal caregiving* [Gender Impact Assessment No. 7]. Retrieved from whv.org.au.

In: Ageing and Mental Health: Global Perspectives
Editors: Wendy Wen Li, Sherry M. Cummings et al.
ISBN: 978-1-63484-777-3

Chapter 3

SWITZERLAND: TOWARDS AN INCREASING AWARENESS OF OLDER PEOPLE'S MENTAL HEALTH

Elizabeth Galleguillos *
University of Lausanne, Switzerland

ABSTRACT

In Switzerland, there is strong evidence of the significant human, social, and economical consequences of mental health problems. For example: mental disorders dramatically increase the risk of suicide and recent OECD estimations demonstrate that direct and indirect costs of mental health troubles represent 3.2% of the GDP. It is not surprising then, that mental health is receiving increasing attention. Despite a performing healthcare system, the federal structure and subsidiarity characterising the Swiss political system tend to impede the implementation of coherent mental health policies. Although the country has one of the highest life expectancy in the world, with over 17% of the Swiss population being over 65, interest in mental health in later life is lacking. This chapter provides an overview of mental health in old age in the context of Switzerland. Without claiming to be exhaustive, it presents information about relevant points such as Swiss cultural specificities, the prevalence of some important mental disorders affecting the elderly, the services available, the role of caregiving, and some recent policy developments.

Keywords: Switzerland, mental health, mental disorders, old age, elderly, subsidiarity

CONTEXT

Located in Central Europe, Switzerland is a non-member of the EU. The Confederation regroups a federal state, 26 cantons and 2 352 communes. There are four official languages: German, French, Italian, and Romansh. With a population of 8 039 060 (Office fédéral de la statistique, 2013) and 591.85 billion CHF of GDP (http://www.bfs.admin.ch), Switzerland is

* Corresponding author: Elizabeth Galleguillos, the University of Lausanne. Email: Elizabeth.Galleguillos@unil.ch.

among the world's wealthiest countries. Federal state regroups the Swiss government (a seven-member executive named Federal Council), a symmetric bicameral Parliament (the States Council, representing the cantons, and the National Council, representing Swiss people), and the Federal Supreme Court. A major feature of its political system is subsidiarity, a constitutional clause attributing "all tasks to cantons unless explicitly delegated to the central state." (Linder and Vatter, 2001, p. 95). Thanks to this, cantons have substantial powers in many important areas, including healthcare and mental health. Federal state must ensure compliance with the existing federal legal framework, such as the federal health insurance law of 1994, named LAMal.

Switzerland, like other industrialised countries, has experienced rapid socioeconomic and sociodemographic changes that have impacted on people's health and quality of life. The Swiss population lives longer and is in better health than in the past (Seematter-Bagnoud, Paccaud and Robine, 2009). The "aged" Swiss residents, that is people of 64–65 and over (i.e., the age when state pension starts to be paid) have benefited from important improvements regarding their health and financial conditions (Oris and Remund, 2012). Such positive changes, however, contrast with the increasing mental health problems the country is reporting (Perrig-Chiello, 2007).

A major shift has been the rapid demographic growth. The Swiss Federal Statistical Office (Office fédéral de la statistique, 2013) reported that between 1970 and 2010 the Swiss population increased by 25%. There have also been important structural changes in its composition. While the number of people aged over 79 has more than tripled, the population under the age of 20 has fallen by 15%. At the same time, the average number of children per woman has decreased from 2 to 1.53[1]. Currently women and men comprise respectively 50.6% and 49.4% of the population, and the proportion of people aged over 64 is 17.4%. Indeed, with an average life expectancy at birth of 82.6 years (84.7 women versus 80.5 men)[2], Switzerland has one of the highest life expectancies in the world. Between 2000 and 2010, life expectancy at birth rose by 3.3 years for men and 2 years for women. Moreover, the Swiss population has a long life expectancy of "good health" (i.e., an indicator based on mortality databases and researches on self-reported state of health within age groups): 70.3 years in the case of women and 69.4 in the case of men[3] (Office fédéral de la statistique, 2012; 2013).

Equally remarkable has been the growth of migration. Between 1970 and 2010 the proportion of foreigners has increased by 76% (Office fédéral de la statistique, 2012). Currently, they represent 24% of the total population, most coming from the European Union (EU) and from European Free Trade Association (EFTA) countries (together, 63.7%)[4] (Office fédéral de la statistique, 2013). Between 1980 and 2008 the number of foreigners aged of 65 to 75 has increased by 209%, and people aged over 79 by 131% (Kasprzycki, 2010). However, the proportion of foreigners decreases dramatically within the aged groups (+64). People aged over 64 represent 7.8% of the foreign population, versus 20.7% of the general

[1] Figures for 2012. Available from: http://www.bfs.admin.ch/bfs/portal/en/index/themen/01/06/blank/key/02/05.html.

[2] Figures for 2012. Available from: http://www.bfs.admin.ch/bfs/portal/fr/index/themen/14/01/key.html.

[3] Figures for 2007.

[4] Figures for 2012.

Swiss population[5]. As a matter of fact, the foreign population increases faster than the Swiss-nationality one (+76% versus +18% during the 1970–2010 period), while the proportion of older migrants remains small (Office fédéral de la statistique, 2012).

Cultural Context

Healthcare governance, the prevalent approach to health, and perceptions of old age have deeply shaped the current perspective of mental health in later life. Regarding the governance of healthcare, it should be noted that subsidiarity has not only affected the division of responsibilities between the three governmental levels, but also between state and civil society. Given the lack of public provisions, family has had the moral and legal duty to take care of their sick, older relatives (Commission d'étude pour les problèmes de la viellesse, 1966; Gilliand, 1988). Still, it was expected that individuals could provide for their own old age through a lifetime of work and private savings, as well through the avoidance of unhealthy lifestyle habits (Commission d'étude pour les problèmes de la viellesse, 1966). In addition, private initiatives have been privileged to the detriment of public interventions (Cattacin, 2006), giving private welfare organisations a crucial role in the provision of health and mental care. Public assistance, developed autonomously by cantons and communes, occurred only in cases of extreme need. Against this background, thus, mental health and mental health problems in later life have been long considered a private issue. To some extent, this approach is still noticeable in contemporary Swiss society.

Mental health has been also influenced by the prevailing curative medical focus of the 20th century (Achtermann and Berset, 2006). Although, since the 1980s—a decade marked by spiralling healthcare costs, important medical progress, and the emergence of chronic diseases such as HIV—the curative approach to care started to be questioned. The country became closer to WHO discourses, and health has been gradually understood holistically, including physical, social, and mental wellbeing. Also, Switzerland adheres to the notions of "public health" and "health promotion" as developed in the Ottawa Charter (Office fédéral de la santé publique, 2007). As noted by Lucas (2010), healthcare moved towards a model more focused on *prevention* and *promotion*; although the former has been privileged to the detriment of the latter. In agreement with the WHO motto "no health without mental health" (WHO, 2001), interest on mental health progressively increased. Presently, the Swiss Health Observatory (Obsan) defines mental health (in French, "santé mentale" and "santé psychique" are two terms equally used, literally meaning "mental health" and "psychic health") as a "dynamic process" including subjective wellbeing, self-actualisation, self-confidence, the capacity to interact with others, the ability to manage daily life, and the capacity to work (Schuler and Burla, 2012). It is agreed that mental health is related to genetics and social and environmental factors, as well as an individual's capacity to mobilise internal and external resources (Office fédéral de la statistique, 2012). There is no particular definition of mental health in old age. Mental disorders are generally defined following the International Classification of Diseases (ICD-10, WHO, 1993) and the Diagnostic and Statistical Manual of Mental Disorders (DSM-IV, American Psychiatric Association, 1994). In recent years,

[5] Figures from 2013. Available from: http://www.bfs.admin.ch/bfs/portal/fr/index/themen/01/02/blank/key/alter/nach_staatsangehoerigkeit.html.

however, there has been a greater awareness about the limitations of these labels, notably among the Federal Office of Public Health (FOPH) (Schuler and Burla, 2012).

Stigmatised views of mental disorders and the mentally ill remain present (Weil, 2009). Regarding the elderly, these stigmas converge with the well-rooted negative images attached to old age and ageing. First, as stated by Ludwig, Cavalli and Oris (2014), "[f]rom the 1930s until the 1970s, the growing proportion of old individuals has been perceived as a social threat" (p. 240). Furthermore, as Perrig-Chiello and Künzler (2013) notice, mental health in later life is still surrounded by "taboos, underestimated aspects and strong prejudices" (p. 2). In Switzerland, as in other western European societies, old age has been historically considered a process of decline (van Dyk, 2014), mental health troubles are often considered a "normal" (p. 94) part of ageing. This view is observed within different segments of society, including healthcare professionals and policy-makers. Also, it is stated here that the tendency to approach old age from an economic angle contributes to a certain alarmism, and over-emphasises the monetary cost that the elderly represent for the healthcare system. This fact, combined with the curative approach prevailing in mental health, could explain why most of the current debate on mental health in later life is absorbed by the question around the financial implications of elderly's mental diseases.

PREVALENCE

The OECD (2014) estimates that the direct and indirect cost of mental health troubles represents 3.2% of the Swiss GDP (i.e., lost productivity, health care costs, and social spending)[6]. However, there is no comprehensive national data on mental disorder prevalence, and there is very little information available regarding the elderly. For example, data about lifelong intellectual disabilities among older people are a void in the Swiss panorama (Institutions sociales suisses pour personnes handicapées, 2011). This section presents information about five mental troubles: Psychological distress, depression, alcohol abuse, cognitive impairment and dementia. It also provides selected data of suicide.

Psychological Distress (PD)

PD is an indicator of psychological wellbeing used on the Swiss Health Survey (SHS) *2012*. It is based on a short, 5-item version of the Mental Health Inventory (MHI-5) and degrees range between "severe," "moderate" and "weak." The SHS 2012 estimates that 5% of the population suffers from severe PD, 13% from moderate PD, and that women present higher rates than men (21% and 15% respectively). Of people over 74, 18% suffer from moderate to severe PD, slightly above the younger population (15–24, 16%). Indeed, the proportion of people with PD increases with age only in the case of men among the age group 25–64. By contrast, there are marked differences following individuals' level of education. People with lower levels of education exhibit higher rates of PD. Among people reporting moderate or severe PD, 29% have an elementary school degree, and 14% a university degree. There are also important regional variations: PD is more frequent within Italian (25%) and

[6] Figures for 2010.

French (23%) speaking cantons than in German-speaking ones (16%). Similarly, important disparities are observed among individuals nationally. If Swiss people and migrants from the Northern and Western Europe show similar rates (17% and 16% respectively), there are marked differences comparing to South-Western Europe (29%), Eastern and Southern Europe (26%) and the Extra-European (25%) population (http://www.portal-stat.admin.ch/sgb2012/; Storni, Kaeser and Lieberherr, 2013).

Depression and Depressive Symptoms (DS)

Depression is not only recurrent, but frequently people with depression suffer simultaneously from other physical or/and mental disorders (comorbidity). DS are measured following a 4-item version of the Geriatric Depression Scale (GDS), and range from mild, moderate and severe. Based on the SHS 2012, around 6% of the Swiss population suffers from depression; although Baer, Schuler, Füglister-Dousse and Moreau-Gruet (2013) point out that the proportion is underestimated since the research does not include people living in institutional settings, such as nursing homes (p. 25). The same research found that, in comparison to men (6%) and the elderly (3%), women (7%) and young people (10%) exhibit higher DS rates (Office fédéral de la statistique, 2014). As a matter of fact, prevalence of mild DS and "negative emotions" (the latter, being a SHS 2009 indicator measured by the question: "How frequently do you generally experience the following emotions: Feel 'blue,' hopelessness, anxiety, depression?" and which answers range in a scale between 0 = never and 10 = always) increases somewhat after the age of 64 (Baer et al., 2013, p. 33). Still, considering the results of the Swiss Survey on Old People Living in Institution (SSOPLI), depression prevalence is high among those aged 65 and over living in nursing homes. Of these, 28% have been diagnosed with depression and 34% report DS, although they have no diagnosis. The percentage of people with neither diagnosis nor DS is 38. In nursing homes, there is no significant variation within age or sex (Kaeser, 2012). Based on the SHP 2009, severe depression is twice as high among migrants, wherein women present higher rates (38.8% and men 20.7%). The SHS 2007 found that within the female population, 4.9% of migrants report DS, compared to 2.7% of Swiss women. It seems that education is a factor contributing to these disparities (Baer et al., 2013, p.35), having also a strong impact in later life. Among the general population aged between 35 and 64, 7% of people with an elementary school degree suffer from chronic depression. The rate is 2.5% among people with a university degree. Of those aged over 65, 5.3% of people with lower educational levels suffer from depression, compared to only 2% of people with higher educational level. Similar trends are found using the 'negative feelings' indicator on the SHP 2009. Among those aged 65 and over, 15% of people with low educational level report negative feelings, this proportion drops to 3–3.7% among people with higher educational level (Baer et al., 2013, p. 35).

Alcohol Abuse

It has been estimated that alcohol dependence affects 250 000 individuals in Switzerland (Kuendig, 2010), although the 2013 rate of alcohol consumption corresponds to the European average of 8.3 litres of pure alcohol per capita (Régie fédérale des alcools, 2014). Alcohol use is common among the Swiss population: 89% of men and 78% of women drink alcohol. The SHS 2012 (see http://www.portal-stat.admin.ch/sgb2012/) found important variations regarding the consumption frequency between sexes; 17% of men and 9% of women drink alcohol daily. About 14% of people exhibited a risky drinking behaviour, which includes "chronic and excessive alcohol consumption" (at least 40 grams of pure alcohol) and 'binge drinking' (at least 60 grams of pure alcohol). Daily alcohol drinking increases with age, especially among men; 30% of people over 64 drink every day, men showing higher rates (38%) than women (20%) Without any relevant difference between sexes, approximately 6% of people within the age group of 65–74 have a risky (a daily consumption of 20 grams of pure alcohol for women, and 40 grams for men) and chronic drinking behaviour (Storni et al., 2013).

The 2012 Continuous Rolling Survey of Addictive Behaviour and Risks (CorolAR) research shows important regional disparities on the rates of daily alcohol consumption. In the Italian-speaking canton (Ticino), 21.8% of people consume alcohol daily, compared to 15.4 in French-speaking cantons, andonly 8.1 in Swiss-German cantons. Here again, educational level seems to have an impact on risky drinking behaviours. Higher rates are found among people of both sexes with higher levels of education, especially among individuals under the age of 35 (Gmel, Kuendig, Notari and Gmel, 2014).

Cognitive Impairment (CI)

CI is used as an indicator of cognitive decline. It is considered that people with CI should present at least one of the following symptoms: altered decision-making capacity, problems with short-term memory, disorientation regarding time or place, difficulty understanding problems, and difficulty communicating and understanding. Data on CI prevalence is only available for the elderly living in nursing homes. Without any relevant difference between sexes and age groups, 59% of this population exhibits at least one CI symptom. Altered decision-making capacity is the most frequently reported trouble, affecting 54% of the elderly. Short-term memory problems affect 46% of the elderly, without any difference between sexes. These problems increase with age, affecting 29% of people aged 65–74, 41% of those aged between 75–84 and half of those over 84. The third most important CI problem is disorientation to time and space, affecting 40% of the elderly. The proportion is higher among the oldest, rising to 44% for the group aged over 84.

Dementia

Prevalence estimations suggest that there are currently 116 000 people afflicted with any type of irreversible dementia, although less than 50% have been diagnosed[7]. The annual

[7] Figure for 2014. Estimations are based on existing European prevalence rates. For people over 64, Alzheimer Switzerland uses the study of Hofman et al. (1991), "The Prevalence of Dementia in Europe: A Collaborative Study of 1980–1990 Findings, *International Journal of Epidemiology*, 20(3), pp. 736-748. For people under 65: Harvey (1998), *"Young Onset Dementia: Epidemiology, clinical symptoms, family burden, support and outcome,"* London, Dementia Research Group of the Imperial School of Medicine.

incidence is 28 000, and resulting costs are estimated at 6.9 billion CHF[8] (Alzheimer Suisse, 2014). By 2030, Switzerland expects 190 000 cases, and 300 000 by 2050–60 (Alzheimer Suisse, 2014; Hanselmann et al., 2013). Among people affected, 65% are aged over 80, and only about 3% are aged 65–69. Under the age of 65, the research estimates that approximately 2 700 people suffer from Alzheimer's. Due to the larger proportion of older women and their higher longevity, it is no coincidence that two-thirds of people with dementia are women. The SSOPLI 2008–09 shows that four out of ten people living in nursing homes have been diagnosed with dementia and most are aged over 74.

Suicide

Epidemiological studies show that Switzerland has an above-average suicide rate as compared to international data, and higher rates than most of the European countries (Czernin et al., 2012). About 10% of the population makes at least one suicide attempt during their life (Office fédéral de la santé publique, 2005). Men's rates of suicide triples that of women's (respectively 17 and 5.8 deaths by suicide per 100 000 inhabitants)[9]. This indicates that suicides increase with age, and men aged over 64 exhibit a disproportionate risk (Office fédéral de la statistique, 2012; Perrig-Chiello and Künzler, 2013).

Services

There are significant regional disparities regarding available services for the elderly with mental problems. Available services include medical and nonmedical care, provided in home or any kind of setting, for a short or a long period. In all cases, care is provided by private and public actors. It takes place in inpatient (hospitals, psychiatric hospital, psychiatric clinics, nursing homes, residential homes) or outpatient settings (outpatient departments of hospitals and psychiatric hospitals, special services of nursing homes, independent practices, and independent services of nonmedical professions). A distinction is made between nursing homes and residential homes. Nursing homes provide both medical and nonmedical services, while the second only provides nonmedical care. There are also intermediary care structures providing day services and emergency short-term services (<24h). Intermediary structures also include sheltered housing that provides medical and nonmedical long-term care (LTC) for dependent elderly. Most of the home-based care (medical and nonmedical) is provided through a home-care service structure called *Spitex* (acronym for the German name "Spitalexterne Hilfe und Pflege"), although there are also professionals working independently such as independent nurses.

Lastly, there is palliative care, which may include medical, nursing, psychological, social, and spiritual support. However, there is no nationwide system of palliative services (see section 5).

[8] Figure for 2009.

[9] Figures for 2011. Data available from: http://www.bfs.admin.ch/bfs/portal/fr/index/themen/21/02/ind32.informations.70301.3201.html.

MENTAL HEALTH SERVICES AND SUPPORT

Aged people with mental health problems may attain services through the Mandatory Basic Health Insurance (MBHI). Regulated through the LAMal, the MBHI is a mandatory federal programme which obliges residents to purchase health insurance. It covers the cost of basic physical and mental illness. While acute and post-acute services are largely covered by the MBHI, LTC is partially excluded. This results in high rates of LTC out-of-pocket spending compared to OECD countries: About 60% of LTC related costs are paid by users (Colombo, Llena-Nozal, Mercier and Tjadens, 2011; Weaver, 2012). In-kind nursing care at home or in institutions is universally provided through the MBHI, but only if prescribed by a doctor. Insurers set the number of hours of nursing home-care services they refund. There are public contributions to services providers. About 45% of home-care services are publicly funded. MBHI covers about 38%, and the rest is covered by patients and other minor sources (Office fédéral de la statistique, 2012). Food and board in nursing homes and residential homes are not covered, just nonmedical home-care such as assistance with the Activities of Daily Living (ADLs) and Instrumental Activities of Daily Living (IADLs). Nonmedical treatments, such as services provided by psychologists and psychotherapists, both considered nonmedical professions, are covered by the MBHI only under medical prescription. Ambulatory medical care is covered by the MBHI only in the case of diagnosed mental sickness; it also needs to be prescribed by a doctor. Alternative or complementary nonmedical treatments for mental troubles, such as art and music therapy, are not included in the MBHI benefits, and only partially covered by some complementary insurance plans.

There are a number of other government services provided which may support older Swiss people. These are connected to the state pension scheme, the Old Age and Survivors Insurance (AHV/AVS). The Supplementary Benefits pension is a means tested supplement for low-income retirees. The Allowance of Impairment is an income-independent allocation for retirees with permanent limitations and needing assistance for ADLs and IADLs, ranging from mild to severe. The AHV/AVS auxiliary equipment benefit covers the cost of auxiliary equipment required for housing adaptation for disabled elderly. Additionally, insured people caring for a dependent elderly relative may claim a bonus which could be taken into account for the calculation of their AHV/AVS pension. There are a number of services available for those older Swiss suffering dementia. *Diagnosed* individuals are typically followed up by a general practitioner (GP) and one of the 39 memory clinics existing across the country (Hanselmann et al. 2013). They can also receive day care in nursing homes and day clinics, since both offer rehabilitation programmes for elderly with mental problems, especially with dementia. People are also administered cholinesterase inhibitors or memantine hydrochloride, each drug treatment being refunded by the MBHI. Drug therapy combining these two drugs is rarely prescribed and not refunded by the MBHI (Hanselmann et al. 2013). There is currently a debate about the inappropriateness of long-term treatment with neuroleptic prescribed to individuals with psychotic disorders (Lustenberger, Schüpbach, von Gunten and Mosimann, 2011). In this regard, Alzheimer Suisse alerts about the side effects of these drugs, and states that about 70% of people with dementia living in nursing homes are treated with this drug (Alzheimer Suisse, 2014).

In terms of nonmedical care, public structures rarely offer specific services for people with dementia. However, the service is widely developed within private organisations

(Hanselmann et al. 2013). Indeed, it is commonly agreed that public programmes, including MBHI, cover only a small part of the needs required by people with dementia and their families. Non-governmental organisations active in the field of old age and dementia, such as Pro Senectute and Alzheimer Switzerland offer a wide range of respite services through local groups. Nonetheless, their range of services varies among regions.

Caregiving

In this chapter, caregiving is understood as a multifaceted concept. It refers to the assistance provided to an elderly person with a chronic mental or cognitive impairment aiming to maintain certain level of independence, health, and wellbeing. In the context of Switzerland it includes a wide variety of (nonmedical) help such as assistance with ADLs and IADLs, financial aid, emotional and affective support, and other instrumental activities or hands-on assistance (Whitlatch and Noelker, 2007). The assistance can be provided in the elderly's home or in institution. Home-care is generally viewed as the most suitable form of caregiving. Duration ranges from temporary to long-term help and may consist of a few hours a week to full daily support. Elderly with mental health disorders often need day-to-day assistance. *Formal caregiving* refers to paid services provided by professionals from public, voluntary and commercial organizations. *Informal caregiving* refers to the assistance provided by family members, relatives, friends and neighbours; it is generally unpaid. Informal caregiving should be understood not only in reference to subsidiarity (section 1.2) but also in reference to the gendered division of labour among the state, family and market. Such setting refers to the "male bread-winner model," i.e., "the model provided for a male family breadwinner to secure the family's income on the basis of his gainful employment and for his wife, who was not in gainful employment, to look after the housework and family support and care" (Eichler and Pfau-Effinger, 2009, p. 623).

In Switzerland, the use of caregiving depends on many factors. These may include financial resources, since nonmedical services are paid out-of-pocket and are not covered under the MBHI; the size and proximity of family, friends and neighbours networks, which are likely to provide informal caregiving; the locality in which the elderly lives, since accessibility to formal community services vary importantly over regions; or still the elderly's and relatives' knowledge and understanding of the offer. Since there is a multitude of public/private payers and providers, it can be difficult to get an overview of the whole "mental health system" (i.e., the range of mental health services available in a given region).

Informal Caregiving

Due to a general improvement on health status and increasing life expectancy, most of the elderly live independently for a long time. Despite no comprehensive data concerning the prevalence of caregiving, research commissioned by the Obsan provides valuable information (Höpflinger, Bayer-Oglesby and Zumbrunn, 2011). Their study confirms that dependency risk (that is, to suffer impairments that impede the realisation of ADLs) increases at the end of the life, concretely over 84. Also, the prevalence is higher among women: About 1.4% of people aged 65–69 needs care (1.7% women, 1.1% men). Within the age group of 70–74, the prevalence is 3.5% (3.6% women, 3.4% men), 6.3% for the group of 75–79 (women 5.7%, men 7.2%), and 13.3% within the group of 80–84 (women 15.9%, men 9%). After 84 the proportion is close to 34%. It is assumed that over 89 the trend reaches 50%, but data is particularly lacking for this age group. It means that there are approximately between 115 000 and 119 000 dependent elderly. Projections estimate that the number of elderly dependents will be between 170 000 and 230 000 by 2030.

The role of informal and unpaid caregivers is particularly important in Switzerland, where nonmedical care remains a "private issue" (Lucas, 2010). As shown in section 3.1, caregiving is far from being fully covered by welfare state programmes, and some tasks (nonmedical ones) are infrequently transferred from family to public or private sector. Although the figures do not specifically refer to the elderly with mental problems, research by Höpflinger et al. (2011) provides some helpful insights about informal caregiving in later life. Following their findings, it is not uncommon for the elderly receive care from more than one person. Often, informal caregivers are direct family members: A third of them are partners, mostly wives. Children also sometimes provide care, but in a different way depending on their sex. Firstly, daughters are much more active than sons in the care of their parents. Secondly, while daughters (and other female relatives) tend to perform domestic tasks and personal care, males mainly help the elderly in their administrative tasks. Finally, it appears that neighbours also participate in caregiving and provide care to elderly dependents living in private households (Höpflinger et al., 2011).

Against this background, informal caregiving has progressively become more visible, and has brought greater awareness to a number of consequences. Caregivers (mostly women) leave the labour-market during a prolonged period to assist a relative, with a consequent loss of professional and human skills (OECD 2005), as well as increased risk of poverty. In Switzerland, there is also a long-term effect because, as in most of the welfare states, social rights are connected to a "continuous job history in standard employment." (Pfau-Effinger, 2011, p. 2). This occurs within the second pillar of the pension system that is occupational. A large proportion of informal caregivers are aged and caregiving demands can negatively affect their own health. Informal work, which includes domestic tasks and care for a family member, is still conducted by those over 64, especially women. Women aged 65–74 spent 27.5 weekly hours performing these tasks, while men spent 19.1. Women over 74 spent 20.5 hours and men only 15 (Schön-Bühlmann, 2010).

Caregiving could represent a burden for those having multiple family duties, such as taking care of more than one relative (partner and grandchildren, for example) and/or maintaining a paid activity outside home.

Formal Caregiving

It is hard to know the volume of professional caregiving allocated in the care of elderly with mental health problems. We know, however, that in 2013, 75% of people receiving homecare (here, each "service" provided is counted as an individual) were aged over 64, about half of them over 79, and two-thirds were women (Lazzeri, 2014).

Among the 1,566 providers, 579 are organisations from the non-profit sector, 694 independent nurses and 293 for profit companies. About 35% of the services provided are nonmedical. Among the 41,866 people working for homecare service agencies, 15,611 people have no educational degree, and 34% of these workers have neither a degree nor any specific training. These people are those performing most of the personal care (such as personal ADLs and IADLs) and domestic tasks (Lazzeri, 2014). Another salient feature is that a huge proportion of these workers are women, who constitute 90% of the workforce (Conseil fédéral, 2007). These low-skilled workers are, most of time, poorly paid and have precarious work contracts. As the Federal Council agreed, their work is "socially undervalued" (Conseil fédéral, 2007, p. 15). In recent years, informal caregiving in the context of dementia has received increasing attention. 98% of the so-called "companion services" (i.e., companionship and supervision) are provided by a family member (Alzheimer Suisse, 2014). Again, most of these informal caregivers are aged women (Hanselmann et al., 2013, p.13). It should be noted that homecare agencies from the public sectors do not propose specific services for people with dementia. There is a greater offer among private companies but the offer importantly varies across the country. Knowing that half of the people with dementia are cared by a relative at their domicile (Alzheimer Suisse, 2014), we can picture the major role played by close relatives. The role of informal caregivers is crucial even if there is good access to home-care. As noted by the Director of a cantonal branch of a non-governmental organisation, home-care is "hardly conceivable without the role of a relative," since he/she ensures continuity of care (JPL, personal communication, September 27, 2011).

POLICY

Mental health policy is not explicitly attributed to federal government by federal constitution. Healthcare and LTC care are both decentralised, and responsibilities lie with the three governmental levels. Cantons are responsible for policy development, implementation, ensuring sufficient levels of provisions within their territory (including hospital and nursing home planning), subsidies, and licensing to service providers. Communes receive delegated implementation powers from cantons, notably with regard to nursing homes, and homecare services. Federal authorities set the legal framework regarding the MBHI, research, education and professional practice, financing, support benefits, and protection of adults (Hanselmann et al., 2013). In 2012, an attempt to increase federal powers in the field of health failed, with parliament rejecting a proposal for a new federal law on health prevention and promotion that could have had a positive impact on the prevention of mental health diseases and the promotion of mental health.

In 1919, the Conference of the Cantonal Ministers of Public Health (CMPH) was founded to coordinate the health ministers of all cantons. Since then, this body has been in charge of handling fragmentation and promoting cooperation between cantons and the central government in the field of health and LTC. Although the CMPH is not a deliberative body, it plays a crucial role in the promotion of more coherent mental health policies, now viewed as an essential aspect of public health.

In 1998, the federal government and the CMPH launched the Swiss National Health Policy Dialogue, a forum of dialogue aiming to promote public health and coordination between federal and cantonal policymakers. It offered the scope to draft a national strategy on mental health, in line with the European trend of promoting cooperative and integrative mental health policies (Lehmann, 2004). Within the forum, the Obsan was created, with a branch focusing on mental health. From 2003, the Obsan was commissioned with the first report on national mental health, with the aim of offering an overview of needs and of setting out national priorities (Rüesch and Mantoni, 2003). Until now, two other reports have been published, in 2007 and 2012 (Schuler and Burla, 2012; Schuler, Rüesch and Weiss, 2007).

Federal government and cantons are currently making considerable efforts to promote a multi-sectoral approach to health, including mental health. Such approach, seen as an essential condition in mental health promotion and prevention, aims to enhance cooperation between all bodies involved in mental health care: federal government, cantonal and communal governments, statutory agencies, private for-profit actors, private not-for-profit and voluntary organisations (Institutions sociales suisses pour personnes handicapées, 2013). Important progress was achieved by the creation of the Swiss Mental Health Network in 2011 (Institutions sociales suisses pour personnes handicapées, 2013). The will to promote a multi-sectoral approach has also been stated in the paper *Health2020*, presenting the federal government's policy strategy for the future in the field of health. There is also a strong push to increase efficiency (cost containment and quality of services) of the healthcare system, and the continuation of integrate care expansion. Mental health promotion and prevention is among the stated goals and measures. An extra focus is put on the issue of "mental health in the workplace" (Département fédéral de l'intérieur, 2013, p. 21). Since the Swiss Mental Health Network operates within federal guidelines, their action too is being focused on the same issue of mental health and working life.

Regarding the elderly, it should be noted that important efforts are being made with regard to dementia. In 2009, the National Council unanimously adopted two parliamentary motions asking for a national strategy on dementia. The FOPH and the CMPH commissioned a report drafting a "National Dementia Strategy" (Hanselmann et al., 2013), ending with the publication of the final "National Strategy on Dementia 2014–17." The document stresses the need for a more integrated approach to dementia and the development of services covering *all* needs of patients and their relatives.

Progress is also being made in the field of palliative care. In 2010, the "National Strategy for Palliative Care 2010–12" (Office fédéral de la santé publique and Conférence suisse des directrices et directeurs cantonaux de la santé 2009) represented a federal government and cantonal authorities' attempt to develop palliative care across all healthcare sectors and set the objectives in this field. Urged by the organisation *palliative ch*, the Swiss Society of Medicine and Palliative Care, the "General Guidelines for Palliative Care" were elaborated and published on summer 2014 as a "working tool" for all those involved in the implementation of the "National Strategy for Palliative Care" (Office fédéral de la santé publique, Conférence suisse des directrices et directeurs cantonaux de la santé and palliative ch, 2014). In this context, the FOPH commissioned research dealing specifically with palliative care and mental diseases (Ecoplan, 2014). Here again, crucial importance is given to both incurable sick and dying persons (often referred as "patients") and relatives.

The Swiss Diagnosis Groups system (SwissDRG) was introduced in 2012, in line with the government's aim to enhance cost containment and healthcare quality. Since then, the system of healthcare reimbursing –including psychiatric impatient treatment– has been modified.

A final reform worthy of mention is the new Swiss Law for Adult and Children Protection, entered into force in January 2013. This reform reinforced the self-determination rights of sick people, including people losing their capacity to make decisions (Hanselmann, et al. 2013), as well as advanced directives regarding end-of-life issues.

GAPS

According to the OECD, Swiss "policies and institutions are not addressing mental ill-health sufficiently." (2014, p.27). Before reviewing some key problems specifically related to later life, it appears necessary to recall recent achievements within the Swiss research on old age.

The past few decades have witnessed important improvements in our knowledge of living and health conditions of elderly people (see for example Lalive d'Epinay et al., 2000). These studies notably acknowledge the heterogeneity of the aged population and the falsity of the equation of old age with mental problems (Calasanti, 2003). Ageing does not systematically mean increasing mental problems since only the 'very old' (+80) constitute a 'vulnerable' group regarding *some* specific mental health disorders, such as dementia. Besides diversity among elderly mental health conditions, heterogeneity is reflected in the "differential availability and use of [material and non-material] resources" (Ludwig, Cavalli and Oris, 2014, p. 241). In fact, both economic and social resources impact on people's mental health conditions. Moreover, because inequalities and disadvantages are cumulative across the life course, the interconnection between resources and mental health conditions in later life needs to be seriously addressed.

Despite an "encouraging" environment (i.e., the growing number of aged people and the expected acceleration of population ageing during the next decades; the increased of mental health problems among the overall population, and the consequent financial implications; the government's commitment to improve the efficiency of the healthcare system) the remaining gaps in the field of mental health in later life appear paradoxical. This is particularly unacceptable knowing that the country has one of the most expensive health systems in the world (about 11% of the GDP). The following sections reiterate some of the gaps that need addressing.

A significant problem is the lack of data set of the healthcare system and population health (Colombo et al. 2011; OECD, 2014). This is particularly true for mental health and more specifically for mental health in later life. The fragmentation and decentralisation of the Swiss healthcare system has contributed to this gap and hampered the federal task of providing health statistics. Aware of this, federal government, together with cantonal authorities, the Federal Office of Statistics (FOS) and the FOPH are making considerable efforts to fill this gap. A vast enterprise started in 1992, with the SHS. It collects data about the population's state of health, health behaviours and the use of healthcare services. Regrettably, the survey does not include the elderly living in nursing and residential homes. Indeed, there is only one survey regarding this population, conducted in 2009 (i.e., the SSOPLI). As mentioned in section 2, it is not possible to determine mental health morbidity in later life, or how the elderly manage mental problems (how they use mental health services, for example). Public health investigations should include mental health among the elderly and the collection of comprehensive data including the *totality* of the aged population.

As highlighted in section 3, there are several problems regarding mental health services for the older population. Most are linked to the federal structure and the culture of subsidiarity. First, there are significant disparities on the services supply across the country, especially regarding nonmedical care. Second, public financing of nonmedical care is insufficient. Consequences of the poor coverage of nonmedical care by the MBHI are particularly dramatic in the case of dementia. The lack of publicly funded support for individuals and their families ('companion services') has been suggested as the main source of preoccupation for the relatives of the elderly's suffering from Alzheimer's disease (Lucas, Giraud, Galleguillos and Maggi, 2010). At the same time, the stressful situation generated by the constraints of caregiving could negatively affect an individual's quality of life. A third problem is related to the complexity of the system of provision, which results in confused and patchy services (Lucas et al., 2010). As a consequence, people with mental health problems and their families are not sufficiently empowered since they cannot make informed choices between mental health services. Finally, there is still a large proportion of mental health disorders that remain undiagnosed and untreated (Schuler and Burla, 2012). Efforts are being made in the field of dementia, but should be extended to all other mental troubles, less visible but nevertheless destructive, such as depression.

Conclusion: A Changing Approach to Mental Health in Later Life

There are many other problems that deserve to be mentioned. However, it is the author's view that most of them are related to the current approach to mental health and ageing. It is true that a change is already happening with regard to mental health, and efforts are being made in all sectors to increase sensitivity to mental health problems. However, as attested by recent national and international publications (OECD, 2014; Office fédéral des assurances sociales, 2014), current preoccupations are focused on the high prevalence rate of mental diseases among working-age groups and the rise of the number of disability benefits due to mental health problems (Schuler and Burla, 2012). As people of retirement age are often viewed as 'unproductive' (because they do not perform any *paid* activity) (Calasanti, 2003), they are systematically detached from this debate. If this trend continues, there is a real risk of disconnecting old age from the general discussion of mental health, and mental health in later life will be reduced to old-age diseases such as dementia. Indeed, maybe the most problematic issue in regard to mental health in later life is the general perception of old age. As highlighted in section 1.1, the approach to mental health in later life remains impregnated by stigmas. So maybe the hardest change to do, as suggested by Perrig-Chiello and Künzler (2013, p. 2), is the promotion of a new approach that considers old age as "valuable," as "useful" and as "profitable" as other stages of human life. This approach is worth further reflection since it could provide a means to effectively address the complex issue of mental health in later life.

REFERENCES

Achtermann, W. and Berset, C. (2006). *Les politiques suisses de santé – potentiel pour une politique nationale. Volume 1* [Swiss health policies – potential for a national policy. Volume 1]. Berne: Politique nationale de la santé, OFSP.

Alzheimer Suisse (2014). *116 000 personnes atteintes de démence en Suisse* [116 000 people with dementia in Switzerland]. Yverdon-les-Bains: Association Alzheimer Suisse. Retrieved from http://www.alz.ch/ju/index. php/des-faits-et-des-chiffres.html.

Baer, N., Schuler, D., Füglister-Dousse, S. and Moreau-Gruet, F. (2013). *La dépression dans la population suisse. Données concernant l'épidémiologie, le traitement et l'intégration socioprofessionnelle* [Depression among Swiss population. Data on epidemiology, treatment and socio-professional integration]. Neuchâtel: Obsan.

Calasanti, T. (2003). Theorizing age relations. In S. Biggs, A. Lowenstein and J. Hendricks (Eds.), *The need for theory: Critical approaches to social gerontology for the 21st century* (pp. 199–218). Amityville, NY: Baywood Press.

Camenzind, P. (2013). The Swiss health care system 2013. In S. Thomson, R. Osborn, D. Squires and M. Jun (Eds.), *International profiles of health care systems, 2013* (pp. 119–127). New York, NY: Commonwealth Fund. Retrieved from Commonwealth Fund website: http://www.common wealthfund.org.

Cattacin, S. (2006). Retard, rattrapage, normalisation. L'Etat social suisse face aux défis de transformation de la sécurité sociale [Lagging, catching-up, normalisation. Swiss welfare state facing the challenges of social security transformation]. *Studien und Quellen – Etudes et Sources, 31*, 49–78.

Colombo, F., Llena-Nozal, A., Mercier, J. and Tjadens, F. (2011). *Help wanted? providing and paying for long-term care*. Paris: OECD.

Commission d'étude des problèmes de la vieillesse. (1966). *Les problèmes de la vieillesse en Suisse. Rapport de la commission d'étude des problèmes de la vieillesse (du 16 décembre 1966)* [Old age problems in Switzerland. Report of the Committee of old age problems study (from 16 December 1966)]. Berne: Centrale fédérale des imprimés et du matériel.

Conseil fédéral. (2007). *Stratégie en matière de politique de la vieillesse. Rapport du Conseil federal* [Old age policy strategy. Report of the Federal Council]. Berne: Conseil fédéral.

Czernin, S., Vogel, M., Flückiger, M., Muheim, F., Bourgnon, J.C., Reichelt, M., ...Stoppe, G. (2012). Cost of attempted suicide: A retrospective study of extent and associated factors. *Swiss Medical Weekly, 142*(w13648), 2–10. doi:10.4414/smw.2012.13648.

Département fédéral de l'intérieur (2013). *Politique de la santé: les priorités du Conseil fédéral. Santé 2020.* Berne: DFI.

Ecoplan. (2014). *Palliative Care und Psychische Erkrankungen* [Palliative care and mental sickness]. Bern: Bundesamt für Gesundheit. Retrieved from BB website: http://www.bag.admin.ch/themen/gesundheitspolitik/.

Eichler, M. and Pfau-Effinger, B. (2009). The 'consumer principle' in the care of elderly people: Free choice and actual choice in the German welfare state. *Social Policy and Administration, 43*(6), 617–633. doi: 10.1111/j.1467-9515.2009.00684.x.

Gilliand, P. (1988). *Politique sociale en Suisse* [Social policy in Switzerland]. Lausanne: Réalités sociales.

Gmel, G., Kuendig, H., Notari, L. and Gmel, C. (2014). *Monitorage suisse des addictions: consommation d'alcool, tabac et drogues illégales en Suisse en 2013* [Swiss addiction monitoring: alcohol, tobacco and illegal drugs consumption in Switzerland in 2013]. Lausanne: Addiction Suisse. Retrieved from Monitorage suisse des addictions website: http://www.suchtmonitoring.ch/fr/page/9-7.html.

Hanselmann, V., Coppex P., von Greyerz, S., Leutwyler, S., Duetz Schmucki, M. and Angele, M., (2013). *Stratégie nationale en matière de démence 2014–2017* [National dementia strategy 2014–2017]. Berne: OFSP and Conférence suisse des directrices et directeurs cantonaux de la santé.

Höpflinger, F., Bayer-Oglesby, L. and Zumbrunn, A. (2011). *La dépendance des personnes âgées et les soins de longue durée. Scénarios actualisés pour la Suisse* [The dependency of old persons and long-term care. Switzerland updated scenarios]. Berne: H. Huber.

Institutions sociales suisses pour personnes handicapées. (2011). *Prise de position personnes âgées avec handicap du 22 juin 2011* [Position statement of 22 June 2011 old people with disabilities]. Retrieved from http://www.insos.ch/publications/prises-de-position/.

Kaeser, M. (2012). *Santé des personnes âgées vivant en établissement médico-social. Enquête sur la santé des personnes âgées dans les institutions 2008/09* [Health of old persons living in nursing homes. Swiss Survey on Old People Living in Institution 2008/09]. Neuchâtel: OFS.

Kasprzycki, E. (2010, March). Des étrangers âgés peu nombreux en Suisse [Few aged foreigners in Switzerland]. *Newsletter Démos, 1*, 6–8. Retrieved from http://www.bfs.admin.ch/bfs/portal/fr/index/themen/01/22/nl.html.

Kuendig, H. (2010). *Estimation du nombre de personnes alcoolo-dépendantes dans la population helvétique (Rapport de recherche N ° 56)* [Estimation of the number of alcohol dependent among Swiss population]. Lausanne: Addiction Info Suisse. Retrieved from www.suchtmonitoring.ch/*docs/library/.*

Lalive d'Epinay, C., Bickel, J. F., Maystre, C. and Vollenwyder, N. (2000). *Vieillesses au fil du temps. 1979–1994: Une révolution tranquille* [Old age over time. 1979–1994]. Lausanne: Réalités sociales.

Lalive d'Epinay, C., Christe, E., Coenen-Huther, J., Hagmann, H. M., Jeanneret, O. and Junod, J. P. (1983). *Vieillesses. Situations, itinéraires et modes de vie des personnes âgées aujourd'hui* [Old ages. Conditions, trajectories and lifestyles of old people]. Saint-Saphorin: Georgi.

Lazzeri, F. (2014). Statistique de l'aide et des soins à domicile. Résultats 2012: chiffres et tendances [Statistics on assistance and home care. 2012 Results: Figures and trends]. Neuchâtel: OFS.

Lehmann, P. (2004). *Santé psychique. Projet destiné aux prises de position jusqu'à mi-mai 2004. Stratégie visant à protéger, promouvoir, maintenir et rétablir la santé psychique de la population en Suisse* [Mental health. Project for the position statement until half-May 2004. Strategy for the protection, promotion, maintaining and restoration of Swiss population mental health]. Berne: Politique nationale de la santé publique.

Linder, W. and Vatter, A. (2001). Institutions and outcomes of Swiss federalism: The role of the cantons in Swiss politics. *West European Politics, 24*(2), 95–122. doi: 10.1080/01402380108425435.

Lucas, B. (2010). Trois gouvernements des démences. Les biopolitiques à l'épreuve des réseaux d'action publique locaux [Three governments of dementias. Biopolitics tested by local public action networks]. *Revue internationale de politique comparée, 18*(4), 61–75. *doi:* 10.3917/ripc.184.0061.

Lucas, B., Giraud, O., Galleguillos, E. and Maggi, J. (2010). Politiques d'aide aux malades d'Alzheimer en Suisse. Volume 2, Rapport de recherche, Resop, Département de science politique [Policies helping people with Alzheimer in Switzerland]. Genève: Université de Genève.

Ludwig, C., Cavalli, S. and Oris, M. (2014). "Vivre/Leben/Vivere": An interdisciplinary survey addressing progress and inequalities of aging over the past 30 years in Switzerland. *Archive of Gerontology and Geriatrics, 59*, 240–248. doi: 10.1016/j.archger.2014.04.004.

Lustenberger, I., Schüpbach, B., von Gunten, A. and Mosimann, U. (2011). Psychotropic Medication Use in Swiss Nursing Homes. *Swiss Medical Weekly, 141*(w13254). doi: 10.4414/smw.2011.13254.

OECD. (2005). Long-term care for older people. Paris: OECD.

OECD. (2014). *Mental health and work: Switzerland.* Retrieved from OECD website http://www.oecd-ilibrary.org/.

Office fédéral des assurances sociales. (2014, March, April). Dossier santé mentale et emploi [Special issue mental health and work]. *Sécurité sociale CHSS, 2.* Retrieved from http://www.bsv.admin.ch/dokumentation/ publikationen/.

Office fédéral de la statistique. (2012). *Statistiques de la santé* [Health Statistics]. Neuchâtel: OFS.

Office fédéral de la statistique. (2013). *La population en Suisse* [Swiss population]. Neuchâtel: OFS.

Office fédéral de la statistique. (2014). *Communiqué de presse n° 0351–1401–40 du 18.12.2014 Publication des tableaux standard de l'Enquête Suisse sur la Santé 2012* [Media release n° 0351–1401–40 issued on 18.12.2014. Publication of the Swiss Health Survey 2012]. Neuchâtel: Service de presse OFS.

Office fédéral de la santé publique (2005). *Le suicide et la prévention du suicide en Suisse. Rapport répondant au postulat Widmer (02.3251)* [Suicide and suicide prevention in Switzerland. Report responding to Widmer postulate (02.3251)]. Berne: OFSP.

Office fédéral de la santé publique. (2007). *Prévention et promotion de la santé en Suisse. Rapport répondant aux postulats Humbel Näf (05.3161) et CSSS–CE (05.3230)* [Health prevention and promotion in Switzerland. Report]. Berne: OFSP.

Office fédéral de la santé publique and Conférence suisse des directrices et directeurs cantonaux de la santé (2009). *Stratégie nationale en matière de soins palliatifs 2010–2012* [National Strategy for Palliative Care 2010–2012]. Berne: OFSP.

Office fédéral de la santé publique, Conférence suisse des directrices et directeurs cantonaux de la santé and palliative ch. (2014). *Cadre général des soins palliatifs en Suisse. Définitions dans le domaine des soins palliatifs dans l'optique de la mise en oeuvre de la "Stratégie nationale en matière de soins palliatifs"* [General framework for palliative care in Switzerland. Definitions with the goal of setting a National Strategy for Palliative Care]. Berne: OFSP, CDS and palliative ch.

Oris, M. and Remund, A. (2012). Les conditions socioéconomiques et culturelles du vieillissement en Suisse [Socioeconomics and cultural conditions of ageing in Switerland]. *Sécurité sociale CHSS. 4*, 203–209. Retrieved from http://www.bsv.admin.ch/dokumentation/publikationen/.

Perrig-Chiello, P. (2007). Mental health in Public Health – the necessity of a life-span perspective. *International Journal of Public Health*, *52*(3), 1–2. doi 10.1007/s00038-007-7012-y.

Perrig-Chiello, P. and Künzler, A. (2013). La santé psychique chez les personnes âgées [Mental health among old people]. *Psychoscope*, *10*, 30–31. Retrieved from www.psychologie.ch.

Pfau-Effinger, B., (2011, May). *New social risks to different work-family arrangements in Europe.* Paper presented at the plenary session of the RECWOWE Workshop for Doctoral Students, Lausanne.

Régie fédérale des alcools. (2014). *L'alcool en chiffres 2014* [Alcohol statistics 2014]. Berne: RFA. Retrieved from http://www.eav.admin.ch/ dokumentation/.

Rüesch, P. and Manzoni, P. (2003). *La santé psychique en Suisse – Monitoring* [Mental health in Switzerland]. Neuchâtel: Obsan.

Schön-Bühlmann, J. (2010, March). Les prestations non rémunérées des aînés [Old people's unpaid services]. *Démos*, *1*, 10–13. Retrieved from http://www.bfs.admin.ch/bfs/portal/fr/ index/news/publikationen.html?publicationID=3865.

Schuler, D. and Burla, L. (2012). *La santé psychique en Suisse. Monitorage 2012* [Mental health in Switzerland. Monitoring 2012]. Neuchâtel: Obsan.

Schuler, D., Rüesch, P. and Weiss, C. (2007). *La santé psychique en Suisse. Monitorage* [Mental health in Switzerland]. Neuchâtel: Obsan.

Seematter-Bagnoud, L., Paccaud, F. and Robine, J. M. (2009). *Le futur de la longévité en Suisse* [The future of longevity in Switzerland]. Neuchâtel: OFS.

Storni, M., Kaeser, M. and Lieberherr, R. (2013). *Enquête suisse sur la santé 2012. Vue d'ensemble* [Swiss Health Survey 2012. Extensive overview]. Neuchâtel: OFS.

Trotta, C., Lang, U. and Schneeberger, A. (2013). Mental Health Care Across Two Nations – Switzerland and the United States of America. *Swiss Archives of Neurology and Psychiatry*, *164*(5), 165–169. Retrieved from http://www.sanp.ch/index.php?id=13.

van Dyk, S. (2014). The appraisal of difference: Critical gerontology and the active-ageing-paradigm. *Journal of Aging Studies*, *31*, 93–103. doi: 10.1016/j.jaging.2014.08.008.

Weaver, F. (2012). Long-Term Care Financing in Switzerland. In J. Costa-Font and C. Courbage (Eds.), *Financing Long-Term Care in Europe. Institutions, Markets and Models* (pp. 279–299). London: Palgrave Macmillan.

Weil, B. (2009). Papier de référence "Santé psychique/santé mentale" (approuvé par le Comité directeur le 11 juin 2009). Santé publique suisse. Retrieved from Santé publique suisse website: http://www.public-health.ch/logicio/pmws/publichealth_mental_fr.html.

Whitlatch, C. J. and Noelker, L. S. (2007). Caregiving and caring. In J. E. Birren (Ed.), *Encyclopaedia of Gerontology. Age, Aging and the Aged (2nd edition)* (pp. 240–249). Oxford: Elsevier.

WHO. (2001). *The World Health Report 2001 – Mental health: New understanding, new hope*. Geneva: WHO.

In: Ageing and Mental Health: Global Perspectives
Editors: Wendy Wen Li, Sherry M. Cummings et al.
ISBN: 978-1-63484-777-3

Chapter 4

MENTAL HEALTH AND AGEING: THE UNITED STATES

Sherry Cummings* and Shannon Trecartin
The University of Tennessee, TN, US

ABSTRACT

Like many countries, the United States is faced with an ageing population. As a result of the increasingly aged baby boom generation, the population of older Americans is expected to increase rapidly. The growth of the older population has highlighted the need to prioritise and advance the current health care system. While much attention has been focused on the physical needs of ageing Americans, much less has been considered with regard to mental health. The United States presently values youth, competence, and independence, which perpetuates a culture of ageism. This directly affects the experience of older Americans, not only through their interactions with others in society, but through the development of priorities and goals for services. The present chapter discusses the context of ageing in the United States, as well as the current prevalence of mental illness among the elderly. Policies and programmes related to mental health provision will also be discussed. Finally, recommendations for improvements to the mental health of older Americans into the future will be provided.

Keywords: United States, mental health, ageism, caregiving

INTRODUCTION

The United States of America's older population, those aged 65 years and over,, numbered 43.1 million in 2013. Older adults represent 13.7% of the U.S. population; about one in every seven Americans (Administration on Aging, 2014). Due to the aging of the baby boom generation, the older population is projected to rapidly increase in coming years and to reach 79.7 million by 2040 (a 21% increase). The growth of the older population has spurred

* Corresponding author: Sherry Cummings, The University of Tennessee. Email: scumming@utk.edu.

heightened awareness of the need to enhance health care provision and ensure the solvency of health care funding for all Americans, especially older adults (Berkman and D'Ambruoso, 2015). Much less attention, however, has been focused on the mental health care needs of older adults. Nonetheless, as the number of older adults continues to grow the demand for effective mental health service will further increase. This chapter describes the prevalence of mental health disorders among older Americans and the context and culture that shape policies about, and service provision for, older adults with mental health disorders. Recommendations to enhance the mental health and well-being of the growing population of older Americans are also provided.

CULTURE AND CONTEXT OF AGEING IN THE UNITED STATED

The American society is complex and comprised of people from a diverse array of nations who have immigrated to the United States over the course of multiple centuries. Such peoples invariably bring with them views of ageing shaped by their own cultural background. In spite of this, over time the United States has developed and maintained a predominate culture that highly values youth, independence, competence, and mobility. The ability to decide for oneself, influence observable outcomes, earn income, and maintain freedom of movement are closely associated with younger populations. Baby boomers (those born 1946 through 1964), the largest generation in American history, were originally characterised by a focus on youth and unfettered freedom. Although the early cohorts of the Baby Boom generation have already begun to reach age 65, and later cohorts will soon swell the ranks of the older population, adverse attitudes toward older adults still persist (Wang and Chonody, 2013). Ageism is multi-dimensional and may contain both positive and negative elements. Yet, in general, older adults in the U.S. are perceived more negatively than the young, and society tends to associate being old with undesirable qualities (Cuddy, Norton and Fiske, 2005). Common ageist stereotypes characterise older adults as unattractive, dependent, and lonely. One study of people 60 years and over found that 77% had experienced ageism, such as the assumption of cognitive and/or physical impairments due to age, and more than half of all respondents reported having multiple ageism experiences (Palmore, 2001). While negative ageist attitudes remain, positive images of older adults also co-exist throughout the general population. Studies have found that older adults are often viewed as kind, warm, and dependable (Kite, Stockdale, Whitley and Johnson, 2005).

For most of U.S. history mental health disorders were viewed as a matter of personal weakness and a cause of shame for both the individual and family. As a result, mental health problems were rarely discussed openly and therefore, public awareness of their prevalence and impact remained relatively low. However, in recent decades, multiple factors have increased society's knowledge and understanding of the commonness of mental health problems. In 1994, for example, former President Reagan announced in a letter to the American people that he had Alzheimer's disease (Reagan, 1994), an action that immediately raised the level and frequency of public dialogue about Alzheimer's disease and related dementias. The return of veterans from wars in the Middle East, presenting with a high incidence of post-traumatic stress disorder and traumatic brain injury, has also substantially increased social awareness of the devastating impact that pernicious events and environments can have on individuals‘ psychological well-being.

Overall, growing awareness of the prevalence of mental health disorders in American society co-exists with the persistence of related negative attitudes. Beliefs and attitudes about mental illness consequently help shape the general availability of treatment opportunities, the specific array of treatment choices, and the willingness of individuals with mental disorders to disclose symptoms and seek treatment. Older adults, as compared with younger members of society, are more likely to view mental illness as something shameful and best kept hidden. Elders' perceptions that psychological disorders are dishonorable often inhibit their willingness to discuss mental health symptoms with others (Hooyman and Kiyak, 2011).

Prevalence of Mental Disorders among Older Americans

Mental health disorders present a major challenge to older individuals. Such disorders not only seriously impair quality of life for individual elders, but also create a substantial societal burden. As the number of older Americans continues to rise, so too does the sub-population of those with mental health conditions. It is estimated that 20% of older individuals in the U.S. experience some type of mental health issue, with Alzheimer's disease and related dementias, depression, anxiety, and substance abuse being the most common (Centers for Disease Control, 2008). Although severe mental illnesses such as schizophrenia and bipolar disorder are far less common in the older population, their consideration remains important since they often result in serious functional impairment.

Dementia

Alzheimer's disease (AD) and related dementias represent a significant public health concern in the United States, one that will grow as the population continues to age. An estimated 5.2 million Americans have AD. By 2050 this number is projected to increase by about 9 million, approaching an estimated 13.8 million. This increase in AD prevalence is attributable to the ongoing growth of the elder population, especially the sub-population of those 85 years of age and over in which the prevalence of AD is the highest (Alzheimer's Association, 2014). In the U.S. two-thirds of those diagnosed with AD and other dementias are female. This observation is partially explained by the fact that women have a longer life expectancy than men (Hebert, Scherr, McCann, Beckett and Evans, 2001). In addition to gender there are also racial variations in the prevalence of AD. In absolute numbers, more Caucasians in the U.S. live with AD and other dementias. However, this is due to the fact that Caucasians represent the largest U.S. racial group. African Americans are twice as likely and Hispanics are 1½ times more likely to have dementia than are Caucasians. Many experts assert that prevalence variations between racial groups are primarily due to other health conditions that present as risk factors for AD and other dementias, such as high blood pressure and diabetes, which are more common among African American and Hispanics (Plassman et al., 2007). Because of the amount of assistance required to care for someone with Alzheimer's disease, or a related dementia, throughout the course of the illness,

AD/dementia is one of the costliest chronic illnesses in the U.S. The yearly monetary costs attributable for all individuals with dementia in the U.S. are estimated to be $214 billion (Alzheimer's Association, 2014).

Depression

Depression is one of the most serious mental health challenges facing the older population. Studies in the United States reveal the prevalence of major depressive disorders (MDD) among the older population to be 1 – 5%. The rates of MDD in older age tend to be lower than in early or middle-aged adults. However, the prevalence of depression rises substantially among medically ill older adults. Research indicates that about 12% of hospitalised patients, between 12% and 20% of older outpatients, and up to 48% of nursing home residents experience depression (Djernes, 2006; Zarit and Zarit, 2007). In contrast to the relatively low rates of MDD, older adults suffer from high rates of clinically significant depressive symptoms or "minor depression." Minor (subdromal) depression has been described as a syndrome consisting of clinically significant depressive symptoms that do not meet the full criteria for a major depressive disorder but are severe enough to cause significant distress or impairment (Hegel, Stanley and Areán, 2002). Reported rates of minor depression range from 10% to 25%. Depression in older adults, whether major or minor, has been associated with longer hospital stays, heightened functional impairment, lengthier recovery times, and increased morbidity and mortality. Depression is also one of the leading factors predictive of older adult suicide. Older adults have the highest suicide rate of any subpopulation in the U.S. (Adamek and Slater, 2006). While the national average for suicide is 11.3 per 100,000 persons in the general population, 14.3 out of every 100,000 older persons end their own lives. Prevalence rates are higher still for non-Hispanic white men age 85 and older, who commit suicide at a rate of 31 per 100,000 persons (U.S. Department of Health and Human Services, 2012). In addition to the substantial and, at times, devastating human costs, depression exerts an economic toll. Depressed older adults are more likely to be hospitalised, admitted to emergency rooms, moved to nursing homes, examined by a physician, and prescribed multiple medications (SAMSHA, 2011). As a result, older adults with depression have 50% higher *healthcare costs* than do non-*depressed elders (*Unützer et al., 2009).

Anxiety

Multiple different diagnoses comprise the spectrum of anxiety disorders observed among older adults, including generalised anxiety disorder (GAD), panic disorder, phobias, obsessive-compulsive disorder, and post-traumatic stress disorder. Anxiety disorders are very prevalent among older adults, yet are often overlooked. Anxiety is as prevalent, if not more so, than depression in the older population. Some researchers report that anxiety is up to twice as common as dementia in older adults, and four to eight times more prevalent than depression (Cassidy and Rector, 2008). Anxiety that reaches the threshold of a diagnosable disorder is present in 3.5 to 10.1% of older individuals. Like minor depression, however, sub-threshold symptoms of anxiety are common. Rates of subdromal anxiety range from 20% of community-dwelling elders to 40% of primary care patients (Hegel, Stanley and Areán, 2002). Like depression, anxiety disorders are twice as common in women as men. Again, as is the case with depression, anxiety disorders are costly to both individuals and society. Older adults with anxiety disorders experience greater functional disability, poorer quality of life and often suffer from comorbid depression and/or substance abuse (Zarit and Zarit, 2007). They also incur increased expenses for primary care and hospitalisation. As a result, anxiety disorders have been estimated to cost the healthcare system over $42 billion per year.

Problematic use of substances among older adults is also a growing phenomenon. It is estimated that close to 4% of the older population experiences some type of substance abuse use disorder (Blank, 2009). This number is likely to grow as the next generation of older adults, raised in the 1950s and 1960s, reaches later life. This cohort of older adults, more comfortable with substance use and significantly larger than any previous cohort, is likely to include an expanded sub-group of individuals with a history of substance abuse and dependence (Blazer and Wu, 2009). Older adults' increased vulnerability to the deleterious effects of alcohol presents a serious problem, which is likely to grow. As a result, the number of older adults with a need for substance abuse treatment is expected to rise from 1.7 million in 2000 to approximately 4.4 million by 2020 (Gfroerer, Penne, Pemberton and Folsom, 2003).

The most commonly abused substance by older adults is alcohol (Lin et al., 2011). The prevalence of alcohol use disorders in older adults has been generally accepted to be less prevalent than in younger groups. Blazer and Wu (2009), for example, found that 6.7% of all of adults 65 years of age or older reported alcohol abuse, dependence, or symptoms of dependence with men reporting a higher prevalence of alcohol use (5%) disorders than women (1.4%). Drinking among older adults that does not reach a diagnosable level can still be highly problematic. Data from three nationally representative surveys reveals that 9% to 10% of men and 2% to 3% of women aged 65 and older are heavy drinkers (Merrick et al., 2008). Additionally, a study from the Substance Abuse and Mental Health Services Administration (SAMHSA, 2008) found 6.6% of older adults to be binge drinkers.

Severe Mental Illness

Close to one million older adults in the U.S. are thought to suffer from *severe* mental illness (SMI) and this number is expected to double by 2030. The majority (70%) of these individuals reside in the community and are reliant upon community mental health systems for treatment, support, and assistance (Cohen, 2003). Although the term *severe mental illness* may refer to a variety of mental health disorders, typically illnesses classified as a SMI include schizophrenia and schizophrenia-related disorders, bipolar disorder, major recurrent depressive disorder, and personality disorders. Individuals typically experience the onset of SMIs in their late teens to early twenties and contend with these psychiatric disorders for the reminder of their lives. Older adults with SMI grapple not only with the symptoms and consequences of their mental illness, but also with age-related changes in their physical health, functioning, and social resources. Compared to older adults without mental illness, those with SMI are more likely to have higher levels of psychopathology (Jeste et al., 2003), decreased functional capacity (Palmer et al., 2002; Unützer and Bruce, 2002), and increased medical problems such as cardiovascular and respiratory disease, diabetes, and cancer

(Unützer and Bruce, 2002). Consequently, those with SMI in the U.S. have a life expectancy that is 20 to 25 years shorter than that of the general population (Parks, Svendsen, Singer, Foti and Mauer 2006).

In sum, a significant proportion of older Americans contend with substantial mental health disorders or symptoms. While some of these disorders, such as dementias, typically occur later in life, others develop in early adulthood and accompany individuals into later life. Older adults with some mental illnesses (e.g., Alzheimer's Disease, schizophrenia) often demonstrate more obvious and disruptive symptoms. Others, such as those with depression and anxiety, may suffer silently. Regardless of their duration or presentation, mental health disorders present serious negative consequences for older adults, their family members, and society.

Caregiving for Older People

Over the past 40 years increased longevity among elders and consequent expansion of this population has led to an increasing number of community-dwelling older adults. The majority of these older adults are healthy and live independently. However, as the number of older adults continues to expand, so too does the subset of those who are frail and require assistance. Familial caregivers in the United States provide the majority of care and support for older adults who require practical, emotional, and financial assistance. The growing need for geographic mobility in response to a rapidly changing job market and a constantly evolving mobile array of employment opportunities has profoundly reinforced the modern trend toward expanding geographic distances between the residences of family members. Despite this powerful reality, 85% of all care provided to older adults in the U.S. continues to come from their family members (Alzheimer's Association, 2014). Only 4.1% of all elders in America reside in institutions such as assisted living facilities and nursing homes (U. S. Census Bureau, 2014).

Over 65 million adults in the U.S. (nearly 30% of the adult population) are the caregivers for older family members. Those who provide such care are most often adult children (41%), spouses/partners (38.6%), and other family members/friends (20.4%) (Wolff and Kasper, 2006). Family members report that the primary reasons that their older family requires care is "old age," Alzheimer's disease and other dementias, and/or specific medical conditions such as cancer, heart disease, stroke, and mental illness (National Alliance for Caregiving, 2009). National data suggest that familial caregivers on average contribute 20 hours per week of unpaid assistance to older relatives. This service benefits not only older adults but also society as a whole. Specifically, informal caregivers contribute 17.7 billion hours of unpaid assistance per year, which, in turn, has an annual value in excess of $220 billion (Alzheimer's Association, 2014).

Care to ailing family members in America has been stereotypically viewed as a woman's role and, despite the growing presence of male caregivers, over 60% of familial caregivers continue to be female, with the vast majority of all full-time care provided exclusively by women (Calasanti, 2009). Typical caregivers for an older family member are middle-aged women who work outside the home. It is striking that over 20% of older adult caregivers are themselves 65 years of age and over (Alzheimer's Association, 2014). While most family members willingly take on care for an older relative, the strain of care provision often has negative physical, emotional, and financial consequences. Caregivers are more likely to report their health as fair or poor as compared to their non-caregiving counterparts. Not surprisingly, nearly one-half of female and one-quarter of male caregivers describe this role as physically stressful, and one-third of all caregivers report that their experience of care provision is emotionally stressful (National Alliance for Caregiving, 2009; Alzhiemer's Association, 2014). Once again, racial/ethnic variations have been documented. Both African American and Hispanic caregivers are more likely to report physical health problems than are Caucasians, while African Americans report lower rates of depression than other racial groups and Hispanics report them to be higher (Alzheimer's Association, 2014).

Care provision can also exert a negative impact on caregivers' economic status. Family members often assume financial costs associated with care. Out-of-pocket expenses for caregivers of those with Alzheimer's disease, for example, exceed $36 billion (Alzheimer's Association, 2014). Many family members also suffer lost wages as a direct result of assuming a caregiving role. It is estimated that more than one-third of caregivers leave the workforce or reduce the number of hours worked due to their caregiving responsibilities. Women are more likely than men to shift from full-time to part-time work (23.3% vs. 7.2%) and are also more likely to drop out of the work force altogether (11.8%) than are male caregivers (2.5%). Lastly, reduction in work hours, result not only in lost wages, but also in a decline in contributions to, and subsequent payouts from, Social Security and private pension funds (Lahaie, Earle and Heymann, 2012). In spite of the emotional and financial strain experienced, research also reveals that some caregivers gain a sense of satisfaction and accomplishment from successfully addressing the caregiving challenges they face. Caregivers report that assuming the caregiver role allows them to give back to their older relative and to reconnect with family members (Alpert and Womble, 2014). Still other family members experience self-growth such as increased tolerance for others, improved patience, enhanced empathy, and greater closeness to God as a result of their care provision (Sheridan, 2013).

MENTAL HEALTH SERVICES

Mental health disorders among older adults result in decreased quality of life, increased mortality and morbidity, greater family strain and burden, and expanded health care costs. Untreated older adults with mental and substance misuse disorders utilise health care and incur costs at twice the rate of their healthy counterparts (Bartels, Blow, Brockman and Van Citters, 2005). Effective interventions do exist to address and support elders with mental health disorders and their family members. Such services include case management, psycho-educational counseling, support groups, adult day care for the person with Alzheimer's disease, and evidence-based interventions such as cognitive-behavioral therapy (Cummings and Kropf, 20008). In spite of this, large numbers of elderly individuals in the United States neither seek nor receive effective mental health treatment. A recent report found that persons aged 65 years and over who experience serious psychological distress are less likely to both perceive a need for treatment and to receive mental health services than are younger adults (Karel, Gatz and Smyer, 2012). As a result, almost 50% of those 65 years and over with a mental health disorder have unmet needs for care (Administration on Aging, 2001).

Community mental health centers (CMHCs) and non-profit organisations, funded through a combination of public dollars, health insurance reimbursements and grants, are available throughout the country and most typically provide services for moderate to lower income individuals. While community-based mental health services are provided to those of all ages, specialised services delivered by geriatric specialists are often not available for older adults (Cummings, Cassie and Trecartin, 2015). Private geriatric practitioners such as psychiatrists, psychologists, and social workers, however, do exist in the community and are found most commonly in urban areas. The services of private mental health practitioners are typically funded through health insurance reimbursements. There is, however, a shortage of practitioners with geriatric training. Gerontological experts in the United States condemn the dearth of health and mental health professionals trained to work with older populations (Bardach and Rowles, 2012; Institute of Medicine, 2012). This shortage is due to multiple factors including scarcity of faculty trained in geriatrics and limited student interest in pursuing geriatric specialties (Bardach and Rowles, 2012; Pelham, Schafer, Abbott and Estes, 2012). In response, professional educational associations have developed geriatric competencies for their academic programs. However, in spite of this, the education of geriatric health professionals falls far short of stated demand (Damron-Rodriguez, Lawrance, Barnett and Simmons, 2008.

Older individuals with mental health conditions most typically visit a primary care physician (PCP) and often present with a physical complaint. In turn, older patients who do receive treatment from a PCP are frequently misdiagnosed and under-treated (Administration on Aging, 2001). While older adults have the highest suicide rate of any sub-population in the U.S., research indicates that physicians often fail to recognise the warning signs. Close to one-half of older victims visit their PCPs within one month of their suicide (Luoma, Martin and Pearson, 2002). Older adults themselves often fail to recognise mental health symptoms that they are experiencing. The majority of older adults do not perceive depression to be a medical disorder, but rather believe it to be a normal part of aging: one to be endured rather than treated (Mental Health America, 2014). Functional impairment, social isolation, and transportation problems also create impediments to care (Bartels, Blow, Brockmann and Van Citters, 2005; Knight, 2011).

In addition to community-based treatment by primary care physicians and specialty providers, hospitals and nursing homes also serve as primary sources of mental health services for many older Americans. Mental health conditions are substantially more prevalent among hospitalised older adults, and 60% of elders who are admitted to the hospital possess a co-morbid mental health disorder (Anderson and Holmes, 2005). Inpatient treatment for depression typically involves psychopharmacology. Focusing on nursing home residents, estimates indicate that nearly 80% have a mental health disorder (Becker, Boaz, Andel, Gum and Papadopoulos, 2012), with Alzheimer disease and other dementias being the most common. Mood disorders comprise the second most common mental health condition in nursing homes. As in hospital settings those with mental health disorders who reside in nursing homes are most typically treated with psychiatric medications. Psychiatric experts, however, note the risk of poly-pharmacy from over-reliance on psychotropic medications and argue for increased usage of psychotherapeutic treatments for older adults (Bartels, Moak and Dums, 2002).

Thus, while services to address the mental health needs of older adults and their families do exist, lack of public awareness, elders' hesitancy to seek out such services and the lack of geriatric professionals create substantial barriers to the development of a geriatric mental health network sufficient to adequately address the range of older adult mental health needs.

Mental Health Care Policies

The primary federal policies that impact older adults' access to required mental health care were developed to create social health insurance programs. Two national social insurance programs provide medical and mental health coverage for older Americans. Medicare and Medicaid, which were signed into law in 1965 as part of the Social Security Act, provide health insurance regardless of income for those 65 years of age and over. Medicare provides health insurance to older adults while Medicaid extends insurance to low-income individuals including the elderly. Prior to the passage of Medicare and Medicaid only about one-half of all older Americans had hospital insurance in contrast to 75% of younger adults who were covered primarily through their employers. In that context, health care costs drained many elders' financial resources. In 1965 nearly one in three older adults was poor (De Lew, 2000). Today only 1.5% of older adults are uninsured, and older adults have the lowest poverty rate of any age group (DeNavas-Walt, Proctor and Smith, 2013).

Medicare provides health insurance coverage for over 90% of all community-dwelling older adults in the U.S. (Smith and Medalia, 2014). The primary sources of funding for Medicare include revenue from a payroll tax that is levied on employers and workers, and premiums (monthly fees) paid by recipients for optional aspects of Medicare coverage. Medicare is available to those older adults who have worked the requisite number of years and contributed payroll taxes into the Social Security system, and to the survivors of those covered. Medicare Part A covers hospital, skilled nursing, home health, and hospice care. Elders whose mental health disorder necessitates inpatient care may receive mental health services in a general or psychiatric hospital. While mental health care in a general hospital is not limited, Part A will pay only for a maximum of 190 days of care in a psychiatric hospital. Annual deductibles and co-pays also apply. Part A is funded through payroll taxes (Medicare.gov, 2015).

Medicare Part B and Part D are optional coverage categories. Part B provides for out-patient coverage including services offered by physicians, clinical psychologists, social workers, and other licensed health and mental health care professionals. In addition to medical services, Part B covers psychiatric evaluation, individual and group psychotherapy, outpatient treatment for alcohol and drug use, medication management, partial hospitalisation (a structured program of outpatient psychiatric services as an alternative to inpatient psychiatric care), and one free depression screening per year. Older adults must pay a monthly premium for Part B, a yearly deductible, and 20% of the Medicare-approved amount for services (Centers for Medicare and Medicaid Services, 2014). Not all physicians and mental health specialists accept Medicare assignment due to the low rate of reimbursement for services provided. Medicare Part D provides subsidised medication by enabling individuals to select a drug coverage program that best fits their needs. Like Part B, Medicare Part D is funded through monthly premiums paid by the beneficiary. Although Medicare drug plans are not required to cover all medications, they do cover many of the medications required by those with mental health disorders such as antidepressant, anticonvulsant, and antipsychotic medications.

Medicaid provides basic health care coverage to low-income individuals including children, pregnant women, persons with disabilities, and older adults (Medicaid.gov, 2015). Medicaid coverage extends to 4.6 million low-income elders. The majority of these individuals also receive Medicare coverage. States administer their own Medicaid programs, decide on coverage, and determine the amount of services available. Certain benefits are mandatory, however, including inpatient hospital care and outpatient services. States may also provide optional services such as case management, and psychiatric inpatient care for persons over 65 years of age. Mental health coverage is provided in all 50 states, although the type and extent of mental health coverage varies. Including all age groups, Medicaid pays for half of all mental health care in the U.S. (National Alliance on Mental Illness, 2013).

Taken together, Medicare and Medicaid fund the vast majority of mental health coverage for older adults in the U.S. Notwithstanding this broad federal commitment, numerous gaps in coverage still exist. Since the passage of the Mental Health Parity and Addiction Equity Act (MHPAEA) and the Patient Protection and the Affordable Care Act (PPACA) some of these gaps have been closed. The MHPAEA was passed in 2008 and took effect in 2010. This act requires that health insurance companies that cover mental health and substance abuse services provide this coverage at the same level as general health services. In the past, many health insurance companies limited coverage for mental health and substance abuse services through higher co-pays, fewer inpatient days, limited outpatient visits, and more restricted lifetime dollar limits for inpatient care. The Act applies only to employers with 50 or more employees who offer mental health and substance use disorder coverage. The provision of mental health and substance abuse disorder coverage is not required (Busch et al., 2014).

The Patient Protection and the Affordable Care Act (PPACA), also known as "Obamacare," expands mental health coverage in several ways. First, the PPACA includes mental health and substance abuse services as part of the designated essential health benefits. This means that insurance companies participating in the PPACA marketplace must provide mental health and substance abuse coverage. Second, PPACA applies federal parity protection to mental health and substance abuse coverage for all new individual and small group plans. Third, the act provides federal funding to states that choose to expand their state Medicaid programs to individuals who fall below 138% of the Federal Poverty Guidelines (Beronio, Po, Skopec and Glied, 2013). Thus far, 28 states have chosen to participate in Medicaid expansion. Participating states are required to provide 10 services to Medicaid recipients including mental health care, behavioral health care, substance abuse care, outpatient clinical services, prescription drugs, and hospitalisation.

Conclusion and Future Directions

The number of older adults in the United States, and the sub-population of those with mental health disorders, is escalating at an unprecedented rate. Through ongoing studies funded by governmental and private organisations, researchers have documented the prevalence of major and minor mental health disorders among community-dwelling, hospitalised and institutionalised older adults throughout the nation. These data provide a vital foundation for the development of efforts to effectively address the mental health needs of older adults. Over the past several decades important gains have been made to respond to the needs of elders with psychological disorders. These include: 1) growing awareness of the mental health disorders in the general population; 2) advances in psychosocial and pharmacological treatments for older adults; and 3) enhanced access to mental health services through the passage of new laws establishing and extending mental health parity. While these efforts represent significant gains, much more remains to be done. Ageism continues to marginalise the presence, needs, and gifts of older adults. Active awareness campaigns are necessary to combat enduring ageism, and enhance public understanding of the positive contributions made by older adults to their families, communities and society.

Concurrent campaigns targeted at the removal of stigma associated with mental health disorders are also essential. Multi-faceted interventions aimed at dispelling negative misconceptions and promoting understanding of mental health disorders should be incorporated into general education and promoted through mass media coverage. Increased awareness of mental disorders and the effectiveness of treatment are critical to ensuring that people seek needed treatment. The growing movement to promote the integration of medical and mental health services also holds the potential to substantially advance the recognition and treatment of mental health and substance misuse disorders for all populations, including older adults. Continued policy development that supports the expansion of integrated health care and promotes the education of medical and mental health specialists trained to work in integrated settings is vital.

Beyond these issues, however, looms the challenge of creating meaningful reform to the Medicare system. Projections of insufficient payroll taxes to support the heath care needs of a burgeoning older population coupled with the rapid rise in health care costs in the U.S. necessitate immediate steps towards addressing this growing imbalance, and establishing a secure and stable system that will ensure quality health and mental health care for all older Americans. Such actions must be taken before the financial demands of providing care for a rapidly expanding older population exert unsustainable pressure on an increasingly burdened health care system. Lastly, continued research is essential. In particular, enhanced identification of risk factors for the development of mental health disorders among diverse groups of older adults has the potential to deliver considerable, immediate returns. In the end, we must focus on the development of effective mental health disorder prevention and treatment strategies, rigorously tested and then selectively deployed in light of a solid evidence base.

References

Adamek, M. E. and Slater, G. Y. (2006). Older adults at Risk. In B. Berkman (Ed.), *Handbook of Social Work in Health and Aging* (pp. 149-161). New York, NY: Oxford University Press.

Administration on Aging. (2001). *Older adults and mental health: Issues and opportunities.* Washington, DC: Department of Health and Human Services.

Administration on Aging. (2014). The Older Population. Administration for Community Living. U.S. Department of Health and Human Services. Retrieved from http://www.aoa.gov/Aging_Statistics/Profile/2013/3.aspx.

Alpert, J. M and Womble, F. E. (2014). Coping as a Caregiver for an Elderly Family Member. *Health Communication*, 1-8.

Alzheimer's Association. (2014). Alzheimer's Association Report: 2014 Alzheimer's disease facts and figures. *Alzheimer's and Dementia, 10*, e47-e92.

Anderson, D. and Holmes, J. (2005). Liaison psychiatry for older people—an overlooked opportunity. *Age and Ageing, 34*, 205-207.

Bardach, S. H., Rowles, G. D. (2012). Geriatric education in the health professions: Are we making progress? *The Gerontologist, 52*, 607-618.

Bartels, S. J., Blow, F.C., Brockmann, L. M. and Van Citters, A. D. (2005). *Substance Abuse and Mental Health Among Older Americans: The State of the Knowledge and Future Directions.* Rockville, MD: Substance Abuse and Mental Health Services Administration.

Bartels, S. J., Moak, G. S. and Dums, A. R. (2002). Models of Mental Health Services in Nursing Homes: A Review of the Literature. *Psychiatric Services, 53*, 1390-1396.

Blank, K. (2009). *Older adults and substance use: New data highlight concerns. SAMHSA News, 17* (1).

Blazer, D. G. and Wu, L. (2009). The Epidemiology of Substance Use and Disorders Among Middle Aged and Elderly Community Adults: National Survey on Drug Use and Health (NSDUH). *American Journal of Geriatric Psychiatry, 17*, 237-45.

Becker, M. A., Boaz, T. L., Andel, R, Gum, A M., Papadopoulos, A. S. (2012). Predictors of Preventable Nursing Home Hospitalizations: The Role of Mental Disorders and Dementia. *The American Journal of Geriatric Psychiatry, 18*, 475-482.

Berkman, B. and D'Ambruoso, S. (Eds). (2015). *The Handbook of Social Work in Aging.* (2nd Edition), pp141-150. Oxford University Press, Inc.

Beronio, K., Po, R., Skopec, L. and Glied, S. (2013). Affordable Care Act Will Expand Mental Health and Substance Use Disorder Benefits and Parity Protections for 62 Million Americans. *ASPE Research Brief*, 1-4.

Busch, S., Epstein, A., Harhay, M. O., Fiellin, D., Un, H., Leader, D. and Barry, C. (2014). The effect of federal parity on substance use disorder treatment. *The American Journal of Managed Care, 20*, 76-82.

Calasanti, T. (2009). Theorizing Feminist Gerontology, Sexuality and Beyond: An Intersectional Approach. In V. I. Bengston, D. Gans, N. M. Putney and M. Silverstein (Eds.), *Handbook of theories of aging* (pp. 471-486). New York, NY: Springer Publishing.

Cassidy, K. L. and Rector, N. A. (2008). The Silent Geriatric Giant: Anxiety Disorders in Late Life. *Geriatrics and Aging, 11*, 150-156.

Centers for Disease Control and Prevention and National Association of Chronic Disease Directors. (2008). *The State of Mental Health and Aging in America Issue Brief #1: What Do the Data Tell Us?* Atlanta, GA: National Association of Chronic Disease Directors.

Centers for Medicare and Medicaid Services. (2014). *Medicare and your mental health benefits*. CMS Product No. 10184. Baltimore, MD: U. S. Department of Health and Human Services.

Cohen, C. I. (2003). Introduction. In C. I. Cohen (Ed.), *Schizophrenia Into Later Life* (pp. xiii-xx). Washington, DC: American Psychiatric Publishing.

Cuddy, A. J. C, Norton, M. I. and Fiske, S. T. (2005). This Old Stereotype: The Pervasiveness and Persistence of the Elderly Stereotype. *Journal of Social Issues, 61*, 267-285.

Cummings, S. M., Cassie, K. and Trecartin, S.M. (2015). Community Mental Health Centers. In B. Berkman and S. D'Ambruoso (Eds). *The Handbook of Social Work in Aging.* (2nd ed.) (pp141-150). Oxford University Press, Inc.

Cummings, S. M. and Kropf, N. P. (Eds.) (2008). *Handbook of Psychosocial Interventions for Older Adults: Evidence Based Approaches.* New York: Taylor and Francis, Inc.

Damron-Rodriguez, J., Lawrance, F. P., Barnett, D. and Simmons, J. (2006). Developing Geriatric Social Work Competencies for Field Education. *Journal of Gerontological Social Work, 48*, 139-160.

De Lew, N. (2000). Medicare: 35 Years of Service. *Health Care Financing Review, 22*, 75-103.

DeNavas-Walt, C., Proctor, B. D. and Smith, J. C. (2013). *Income, Poverty, and Health Insurance Coverage in the United States: 2012.* Washington, D.C: U.S. Census Bureau, Current Population Reports, U.S. Government Printing Office.

Djernes J. K. (2006). Prevalence and predictors of depression in populations of elderly: a review. *Acta Psychiatrica Scandinavica, 113*, 372-387.

Gfroerer, J., Penne, M., Pemberton, M. and Folsom, R. (2003) Substance abuse treatment need among older adults in 2020: The impact of the aging baby-boom cohort. *Drug and Alcohol Dependence, 69*, 127-135.

Hegel, M.T., Stanley, M. A. and Areán, P. E. (2002). Minor Depression and Subthreshold Anxiety Symptoms in Older Adults: Psychosocial Therapies and Special Considerations. *Generations, 26*, 44-49.

Hebert L. E., Scherr, P. A., McCann J. J., Beckett L. A., Evans D. A. (2001) Is the Risk of Developing Alzheimer's Disease Greater for Women than for Men? *American Journal of Epidemiology, 153*, 132–6.

Hooyman, N. R. and Kiyak, H. A. (2011). *Social Gerontology: A Multidisciplinary Perspective* (9th ed.). Boston, MA: Allyn and Bacon.

Institute of Medicine, (2012). *The Mental Health and Substance Use Workforce for Older Adults: In Whose Hands?* Washington, DC: The National Academies Press.

Jeste, D. V., Twamley, E. W., Eyler Zorilla, L. T., Golshan, S., Patterson, B. W. and Palmer, B. W. (2003). Aging and outcome in schizophrenia. *Acta Psychiatrica Scandinavica, 107*, 336-343.

Karel, M., Gatz, M. and Smyer, M. (2012). Aging and mental health in the decade ahead: what psychologists need to know. *American Psychologist, 67*, 184-198.

Kite, M. E., Stockdale, G. D., Whitley, B. E., Jr. and Johnson, B. T. (2005). Attitudes Toward Younger and Older Adults: An Updated Meta-Analytic Review. *Journal of Social Issues, 61*, 241-266.

Knight, M. (2011). Access to Mental Health Care Among Older Adults. *Journal of Gerontological Nursing, 37*, 16-21.

Lahaie, C., Earle, A. and Heymann, J. (2012). An Uneven Burden: Social Disparities in Adult Caregiving Responsibilities, Working Conditions, and Caregiver Outcomes. *Research on Aging, 35*, 243-274.

Lin, J. C., Karno, M. P., Grella, C. E., Warda, U., Liao, D. H., Hi, P. and Moore, A. A. (2011). Alcohol, Tobacco, and Non-Medical Drug Use Disorders in U.S. Adults Aged 65 and Older: Data from the 2001-2002 National Epidemiologic Survey of Alcohol and Related Conditions. *American Journal of Geriatric Psychiatry, 19*, 292-299.

Luoma, J. B., Martine, C. E. and Pearson, J. L. (2002). Contact with mental health and primary care providers before suicide: a review of the evidence. *American Journal of Psychiatry, 159*, 909-916.

Medicaid.gov (2015). Seniors and Medicare and Medicaid Enrollees. Retrieved from http://www.medicaid.gov/medicaid-chip-program-information/by-population/by-population.html.

Medicare.gov (2015). *The official U.S. government site for Medicare.* Retrieved from http://www.medicare.gov/.

Mental Health America. (2014). Depression in Older Adults. Retrieved from http://www.mentalhealthamerica.net/conditions/depression-older-adults.

Merrick, E. L., Horgan, C. M., Hodgkin, D., Garnick, D. W., Houghton, S. F, Panas, L., Saitz, R. and Blow, F. C. (2008). Unhealthy Drinking Patterns in Older Adults: Prevalence and Associated Characteristics. *Journal of the American Geriatrics Society, 56*, 214-223.

National Alliance for Caregiving (2009). Executive summary: Caregiving in the U.S. Retrieved from http://www.caregiving.org/pdf/research/CaregivingUSAllAgesExecSum.pdf.

National Alliance on Mental Illness. (2013). *Medicaid expansion and mental health.* Retrieved from http://www.nami.org/Content/NavigationMenu/Inform_Yourself/About_Public_Policy/Issue_Spotlights/NAMI-FactSheet3-Medicaid.pdf.

Palmer, B. W., Heaton, R. K., Gladsjo, J. A., Evans, J. D., Patterson, T. L., Godshan, S. and Jeste, D. V. (2002). Heterogeneity in functional status among older outpatients with schizophrenia: employment history, living situation, and driving. *Schizophrenia Research, 55*, 205-215.

Palmore, E. (2001). The Ageism Survey: First findings. *The Gerontologist, 41*, 572-575.

Pelham, A., Schafer, D., Abbott, P. and Estes, C. (2012). Professionalizing gerontology: Why AGHE must accredit gerontology programs. *Gerontology and Geriatrics Education, 33*, 6-19.

Parks, J., Svendsen, D., Singer, P., Foti, M.E. and Mauer, B. (2006). *Morbidity and Mortality in People with Serious Mental Illness.* Alexandria, VA: National Association of State Mental Health Program Directors (NASMHPD) Medical Directors Council.

Plassman, B. L, Langa, K. M., Fisher, G. G., Heeringa, S. G., Weir, D. R., Ofstedal, M. B., …Wallace, R. B. (2007). Prevalence of dementia in the United States: the aging, demographics, and memory study. *Neuroepidemiology, 29*, 125-32.

Regan, R. (1994, Nov. 5). *Text of letter written by President Ronald Reagan announcing he has Alzheimer's disease.* Retreived from http://www.reagan.utexas.edu/archives/reference/alzheimerletter.html.

Substance Abuse and Mental Health Services Administration. (2011). *The Treatment of Depression in Older Adults: Depression and Older Adults: Key Issues.* Rockville, MD: Center for Mental Health Services, Substance Abuse and Mental Health Services Administration, U.S. Department of Health and Human Services.

Sheridan, M. (2013). Elders caring for elders: the role of religious involvement and spiritual rewards on caregiver stress, resources and health. *Journal of Religion and Spirituality in Social Work: Social thought, 32*, 397-421.

Smith, J. C. and Medalia, C. (2014). *Health Insurance Coverage in the United States: 2013*. Washington, DC: U.S. Government Printing Office.

Substance Abuse and Mental Health Services Administration. (2008). Results from the 2005 National Survey on Drug Use and Health: National Findings. Retrieved from http://www.oas.samhsa.gov/NSDUH/2k5NSDUH/Alts.htm#Fig3-1.

Unützer, J. and Bruce, M. L. (2002). The Elderly. *Mental Health Services Research, 4*, 245-247.

Unützer, J., Schoenbaum, M., Katon, W., Fan, M., Pincus, H., Hogan, D. and Taylor J. (2009). Health care costs associates with depression in medically ill fee-for-service Medicare participants. *Journal of the American Geriatric Society, 57,* 506-10.

U.S. Census Bureau (2014). *65+ in the United States: 2010*. Washington, DC: U.S. Government Printing Office.

U.S. Department of Health and Human Services Office of the U.S. Surgeon General and of the National Action Alliance for Suicide Prevention. (2012). *2012 National Strategy for Suicide Prevention: Goals and Objectives for Action*. Washington, DC: Department of Health and Human Services.

Wang, D. and Chonody, J. (2013). Social workers' attitudes toward older adults: A review of the literature. *Journal of Social Work Education, 9*, 150-172.

Wolff, J. L. and Kasper, J. D. (2006). Caregivers of Frail Elders: Updating a National Profile. *The Gerontologist, 46*, 344-356.

Zarit, S. H. and Zarit, J. M. (2007). *Mental Disorders in Older Adults: Fundamentals of Assessment and Treatment*. New York, NY: The Gildford Press.

In: Ageing and Mental Health: Global Perspectives
Editors: Wendy Wen Li, Sherry M. Cummings et al.
ISBN: 978-1-63484-777-3

Chapter 5

AGEING AND MENTAL HEALTH IN DIVERSITY: A NEW ZEALAND EXPERIENCE

Hong-Jae Park [*] ***and Carole Adamson***
The University of Auckland, Auckland, New Zealand

ABSTRACT

As is the case in most developed nations, a significant proportion of New Zealand's older people experience mental health issues in their everyday lives. This chapter aims to provide an outline of 'mental health and older adults' in the New Zealand context. This background snapshot provides a foundation for the New Zealand landscape on this topic. Cultural initiatives and legislative acts are highlighted alongside current programmes in mental health for older people. Challenges around care for older people with mental health issues abound due to wide-ranging complexities surrounding their care and treatment; there is also limited subject-specific research being undertaken. Urgently needed are new approaches to economic planning, health care and welfare support, retirement policies, innovative living space arrangements and inter-generational relations alongside the promotion of constructive views on ageing.

Keywords: ageing, diversity, mental health, New Zealand

INTRODUCTION

Like other developed nations, New Zealand faces a very challenging time in its health and social care future as its population rapidly ages. Older people constitute a significant proportion of the New Zealand population. An increase in life expectancy is the key factor leading to this ageing phenomenon, along with improvements in mortality rates at all ages. Declines in the fertility rate further contribute to the profile of an ageing population. The Post-World War II baby boom cohort (people born between 1946 and 1964) is generally regarded as the impetus for the rapidly ageing population and has wide social policy

[*] E-mail: hj.park@auckland.ac.nz.

implications. As its population ages, the number of vulnerable people in New Zealand needing social and health care provision increases. This brings further economic and political pressure in relation to the provision of government-funded services. Health care for older people is thus an ongoing challenge that requires considerable coordination of both social and financial resources.

Mental health in older people is of critical importance as growing numbers of older people in New Zealand experience a variety of mental illnesses. It is generally assumed that the prevalence of mental illness continues to increase as people age, and as a result, the costs of providing services and other assistance for this population are expected to rise significantly (Ministry of Health 2011). There have been a range of social interventions to support older people with mental health issues in New Zealand. The government and health authorities provide state-led health and social care initiatives for those people affected by mental disorders or related problems. A broad range of non-governmental organisations (NGOs) also provide care and services to promote the mental health and wellbeing of older people in the community.

This chapter focuses on exploring mental health and older adults in the New Zealand context. It provides a brief snapshot of New Zealand's ageing population, followed by a contextual description of public perceptions both of ageing and of mental health. Discussion then moves to prevalence and the main mental health issues for older people from different cultural backgrounds in New Zealand. This chapter also explores social responses to these mental health issues, covering legislation, policies, and service provision and interventions. In closing, the chapter addresses primary gaps and significant steps to promote the mental health and wellbeing of older people in New Zealand.

Older People in Diversity: A Brief Snapshot

Reaching the age of 65 is a significant milestone in New Zealand. Currently, it is the age at which people are eligible for government-funded universal superannuation (the non-means-tested pension). Despite the fact that there is no official retirement age in New Zealand, this age requirement of superannuation entitlement sends a strong message that people are defined by statute as 'older people' when they reach the age of 65. The 2013 census data show that 607,032 people were aged 65 or over, or 14.3% of all New Zealanders (Statistics New Zealand 2014a). The number of older people is expected to more than double between 2015 and 2050, constituting one-quarter or more of all New Zealand residents. Specifically, the number of people aged 85 and over (the oldest-old group) is expected to more than quadruple, from 73,317 in 2013 to over a quarter of a million by 2050 (Statistics New Zealand 2006).

The ageing population in New Zealand is highly diverse. Within the group of older people, individuals vary widely in terms of age, socio-economic status and health status. In 2013, men were expected to live until age 79.3 years, while the life expectancy of women was 83 (Statistics New Zealand 2014b) resulting in fewer men than women among older New Zealanders. The 2013 census data showed that in this age group, 46% of people were men, while 54 per cent were women. Females also outnumbered males in the group of those aged 85 years and over (64.3%).

Reflecting on other age groups in New Zealand, older people are divided into five major ethnic groups: European, Māori (the indigenous people of New Zealand), Pacific, Asian[1], and other populations. In the 2013 census, most (over 83%) older people identified themselves as European. The number of Māori older people is relatively small at 32,184 (approximately 5.4% of older New Zealanders) although Māori constituted 14.9% of the total population in 2013. Only 5.3% of the Māori population were aged 65 and over, a factor related to the lower age quartile for life expectancy among this group (average of 72 years in 2012). A similar pattern is seen in the Pacific population (people whose origins are in Samoa, Tonga, Niue and other smaller islands). Older people in this group comprised only 2% of all Pacific Islanders in the 2013 census. New Zealand has seen the numbers of Asian residents almost double since 2001, with the largest overseas-born communities coming from China, India, the Philippines, and Korea. The number of Asian older people increased to 27,312 (5.8% of all Asians in 2013), and this increase will continue as the population ages. Other ethnic groups consist of people who identify with Middle Eastern, Latin American or African ethnic groups. These populations are relatively younger than any other ethnic groups, which will continue until the first generation of these groups reach the 'old age' categories.

Living standards for older New Zealanders are slightly higher than those of the population as a whole. Old age poverty is below the average of Organisation for Economic Co-operation and Development countries (OECD 2013). Socio-economic positions, however, vary among older New Zealanders; the levels of income and wealth are significantly different among subgroups. A majority of older New Zealanders remain heavily dependent on New Zealand Superannuation (The New Zealand Superannuation and Retirement Income Act 2001). Approximately 40% of superannuation recipients have no other income, while for the next 20%, the taxable pension accounts for 85% of their income (Perry 2010). Various types of social assistance under the Social Security Act 1964 are also given to some older people. The more recently introduced KiwiSaver is an auto-enrolment pension scheme instituted under the KiwiSaver Act 2006, and is expected to play an active role in boosting retirement income in the future. Other income sources for older New Zealanders include income derived from business, income from rental properties, savings and interest, dividends, trust or estate income, employment, and income earned from overseas (Stephens, Alpass and Towers 2010).

Mental Health Issues among Older People

There is considerable evidence to show that an increasing number of older people experience mental health problems in New Zealand (Ministry of Health 2011). Both growing older and settling into retirement involve a change in lifestyle for most older people, and such a change can cause significant problems in mental health and wellbeing. Major mental illnesses in older age include depression and anxiety disorders, schizophrenia and other psychotic disorders, cognitive impairment, and alcohol and substance-related disorders. In particular, Alzheimer's disease and other types of dementia are common age-related mental disorders among older New Zealanders. Such mental health issues are often associated with 'negative' experiences in older age such as losses and changes in a range of life domains,

[1] The group of Asians here includes both people from South East Asia and East Asia or Asian not elsewhere specified (Statistics New Zealand 2014a).

including physical health, income, relationships, and social participation. There are also associations between some mental health issues and social identities, such as gender, ethnicity or socio-economic status (Dulin, Stephens, Alpass, Hill and Stevenson 2011).

Whilst mental illness crosses all societal boundaries affecting both genders and every ethnic group indiscriminately (Budge, Stephens and Stichbury 2014), there are to date, few New Zealand publications that provide substantial information on mental health issues in older people. Limited research and publications on mental health issues amongst older people in New Zealand hamper data-driven policy initiatives and the development of assessments and interventions. Nonetheless, it can be assumed that since mental health and wellbeing cannot be separated from other determinants of health, mental health challenges in older people may rise as their social and economic circumstances alter with time.

Thus far, a significant longitudinal study carried out by the Health and Ageing Research Team (HART) at Massey University has established that mental health is strongly impacted by the phenomenon of loneliness across both genders and across ethnic groups (Budge, Stephens and Stichbury 2014). The New Zealand Mental Health Survey (Oakley Browne, Wells, and Scott, 2006) showed that the prevalence rate of mental disorders for older people in the community was just over 7%, while 'serious mental disorder' for this age group was at 1.1%. This survey did not include people with dementia or residents in hospital or in assisted living facilities. However, it can be assumed that prevalence rates of mental disorders among these groups would be much higher than those among the general older population in the community (Elliot, cited in Ministry of Health 2011). It could be argued that actual prevalence rates of mental disorders among the whole population of older New Zealanders are of significant concern and this includes people in residential or hospital care (Kuruvilla, Davidson, McCabe, Mellor and Moore 2007).

Dementia

Dementia (as a neurocognitive disorder) is the most common mental disorder that affects a significant proportion of older New Zealanders. In 2011, there were more than 48,000 people affected by dementia; among them, 95% were older adults (aged 65 and over). This number is expected to double by 2025 bringing the number of dementia sufferers in New Zealand to approximately 150,000 by 2050 (Perkins 2013). The most common cause of dementia is Alzheimer's disease (accounting for 70% of all dementia), followed by vascular disease, Lewy body dementia (LBD), front-temporal dementia, and other types of dementia.

Depression

Another common mental disorder is depression in older age. It is estimated that up to 20 per cent of people aged 65 or over are affected by this illness, of which 3 per cent are affected with severe depression (Ministry of Health 2011). Major depression is more common among women than men, and older people from minority backgrounds are particularly vulnerable to this mental illness, suggesting a psycho-social dimension to the experience. Depression is also related to other chronic illnesses including physical disability, heart diseases, anxiety and dementia (see Chapman, Perry and Strine 2005). This mental disorder has been recognised as the most common cause of suicide in older people. Although the rate of suicide for men aged 85 years and older is very high (31 per 100,000 in 2012/13), the link between suicide and mental health is likely unknown (see Harvey 2013). However, studies consistently show that many New Zealand elders live in loneliness and isolation, and are likely to experience various levels of depression during their ageing processes (Budge et al. 2014).

Substance Abuse

Alcohol abuse and other drug disorders also put many New Zealand elders at risk of immediate or future damage to their physical or mental health. Along with high levels of alcohol consumption, maladaptive patterns of substance use may be a significant concern among older New Zealanders. The prevalence of alcohol and substance abuse is expected to increase due to the growing number of 'baby boomer' seniors who are likely to have been exposed to such harmful drugs during their life-span (Khan, Davis, Wilkinson, Sellman and Graham 2002).

Loneliness in old age can also contribute to increased alcohol consumption (Khan, Wilkinson, and Keeling, 2006). It is also assumed that co-morbidity of alcohol and substance abuse and other mental disorders is common, as alcohol and drug dependence can cause serious damage in the brain and other vital organs.

Anxiety and Psychoses

In addition, mental disorders in older people include anxiety disorders (including specific and social phobias), schizophrenia, and other psychotic conditions. These disorders may start in early or middle adulthood and persist through to older age. For instance, post-traumatic stress disorder has been frequently reported among war veterans who served in the Second World War, the Korean War and the Vietnam War (Ikin, Creamer, Sim and Mckenzie 2010; Long, Macdonald and Chamberlain 1996) and New Zealand's continuing military involvement in overseas deployments suggests that this is likely to be an ongoing issue. Whilst intervention and support for those with these disorders may have continuity as they age, isolation, losses and changes in psycho-social and economic circumstances may compound the challenges facing people with pre-existing disorders.

Culture and Mental Health

Mental health is generally determined by a combination of biological, psychological and social factors. However, culture also influences people's beliefs and perception of mental illness, symptomatic expression, and help-seeking patterns. In some cultures, mental health has been viewed as a result of supernatural phenomena where contemporary medical treatments are viewed less favourably than traditional cultural or spiritual interventions. Current perspectives in New Zealand are more centred on recovery-focused medical and psychological interventions through scientific and psycho-social approaches. Therefore, it can be said that cross-cultural variations in mental health models are significant in the New Zealand context where a wide range of cultures, both indigenous and settler, are in existence.

Indigenous approaches to mental health have been a unique feature of New Zealand health services since the early 1980s. The model 'Te Whare Tapa Whā' (Durie 1998) – the four cornerstones (or walls of the house) of health – is the main framework for understanding Māori and their wellbeing and is a model mainstreamed within health and welfare practice within Aotearoa, New Zealand. This model is based on the indigenous perspective of health and wellbeing in the Māori population. Mental health is viewed as one of four developmental components of wellbeing: Taha tinana (physical growth and development), Taha wairua (spiritual essence, strongly held values and beliefs), Taha whānau (family health through belongingness and togetherness), and Taha hinengaro (mental health). The mind and the soul are viewed as not being separable from the body, and therefore both form integral components of health and wellbeing within the context of family and broader belonging. In this holistic framework, mental health is constructed as a component of wellbeing that contributes to, and is dependent upon belonging in family and community, connectedness to the universe, and physical wellbeing. Mental health and wellbeing of Māori in New Zealand is characterised by the positive role that kaumātua (elders) play within Māori society, whereby Māori elders have positive status and actively participate within their communities. Moreover, the efforts of mental health services to provide culturally appropriate service delivery are beneficial for many older people in New Zealand.

Pacific communities in New Zealand, as a diverse group of people, have also developed culturally specific models of health and wellbeing. For example, the Fonofale model of health, created by Pulotu-Endemann (2009), uses the Samoan concept of fale (house) as a metaphor for wellness (Laracy, Trimmer and Love-Gray 2011). The main feature of this model is its emphasis on the significance of aiga (extended family) as the medium of cultural values and beliefs. The role of the community is also considered as essential to promoting health and wellbeing. In this model, four pou (posts) represent different dimensions: spiritual, physical, mental and other factors (such as age, gender, sexuality and socio-economic status). The mental dimension directly relates to the wellbeing or health of the mind, while it is also affected by the sound functioning of other components (Polotu-Endemann 2009).

While Asian migrant populations are rapidly growing in New Zealand, mental health issues for these groups are under-researched. One New Zealand study conducted in 1999 has, however, found that depression is a rising problem among older Chinese migrants in comparison with the general population (Abbott, Wong, Williams, Au and Young 1999). Among Asian cultures, mental illness is often viewed as a lack of self-control involving shame and guilt in family and community contexts (Ho, Au, Bedford and Cooper 2003). This cultural view often contributes to a reluctance to report mental illnesses or to seek help for those problems in the community. Furthermore, difficulties in communication and social engagement may prevent these people from utilising health and social care services in their host society.

Cultural differences in symptomatic expressions of mental health problems further exacerbate the mental health issues found among ethnic minority groups. For example, a qualitative study with Korean-New Zealanders shows that those people experiencing elder abuse and neglect within their family were likely to report self-diagnosed *Hwa-byung* (Korean culture-bounded anger syndrome), that is, they had a greater tendency to present their distress in terms of physical (somatic) rather than mental symptoms (Park 2014).

In addition, mental health in older refugees remains largely under-researched in the New Zealand context. Research has shown that older refugees are vulnerable to a range of mental health issues due to experiences of physical or psychological trauma prior to their resettlement in New Zealand (Gray and Elliott 2001). International studies in this area have also consistently shown that depression and anxiety disorders are very common among older refugees as a result of complex adjustment factors and their sense of isolation. As stated above, the early findings of the HART points to a strong link between mental health and loneliness (Budge et al. 2014). Thus, in tandem with the number of refugees growing older, the prevalence rates of mental illness among these populations are also expected to rise significantly in the near future.

MENTAL HEALTH POLICY RELATED TO OLDER PEOPLE

Since its earlier stage of settlement by Europeans, New Zealand has developed a collaborative model in its mental health system that is operated by three major structural bodies: governmental, regional, and local community organisations.

The Ministry of Health is the government's principal organisation responsible for mental health legislation and policy, as well as the provision of funding for some services. At the implementation level, 20 District Health Boards (DHBs) provide mental health services through local hospitals and other services in their districts across the country. A range of NGOs also deliver health and social care services for people with mental health issues and their families in the community. Most NGO services are funded or purchased by the Ministry of Health and DHBs.

Social responses to mental health issues in older people range from legislative acts, to social policies and programmes, and to practice in health and social services. These responses provide not only prevention programmes, treatment, and intervention, but also serve to ensure protection of the human rights and safety of people with mental illness and other members in the community.

Legislation

Under the current New Zealand government system, the Ministry of Health is responsible for the administration and implementation of mental health legislation and regulations. Legislative acts relating to mental health have consistently evolved to ensure that all services operate appropriately in the current social, economic, and cultural environments. Such legislation also influences how older people with mental illness manage their everyday lives and engage with their whānau (family) and communities. Although there is no specific law focusing on the mental health of older people, the following are some examples of legislation which regulate the provision of involuntary care and treatment in the current legal system.

Firstly, the Mental Health (Compulsory Assessment and Treatment) Act 1992 is the cornerstone legislation that enforces the compulsory assessment and treatment of people who are considered to be 'mentally disordered' (an abnormal state of mind), and to be of serious danger to their own or others' health and safety. The aim of this Act is to define the circumstances in which people with mental disorders are subjected to compulsory psychiatric assessment or treatment. The Act also addresses the human rights of those within its remit in order to provide better protection for their basic rights.

Another important law relating to mental health in older people is the Alcoholism and Drug Addiction Act 1966. The purpose of this Act, which does not specifically refer to older people, is to provide those who are diagnosed as alcoholics and drug addicts with appropriate care and treatment within the community. The Act allows courts to make an order to force those so diagnosed to undergo compulsory treatment at specially certified institutions. In some involuntary cases, those people subjected may feel that their freedom is being threatened because the treatment is compulsory. The effectiveness of this outdated Act has not been well established in relation to compulsory and residential treatment programmes for chronic alcohol and drug addiction (Broadstock, Brinson and Weston 2008).

The Protection of Personal and Property Rights Act 1988 makes provision for people who have lost the capacity to make or understand decisions about their own personal affairs, property or treatment, or who are no longer able to inform others of their wishes. The Act includes the capacity to make advanced directives for those with deteriorating or episodic mental illness.

In relation to the care of vulnerable older adults, the Crimes Amendment Act 2011 deems it an offence to fail to protect those people (such as people with severe dementia) from the risk of elder abuse and neglect. The Act requires family members and caregivers to take appropriate steps when a vulnerable adult in the household is known to be abused or neglected. In any hospital, institution, or residence where vulnerable adults reside, each staff member is also responsible for taking appropriate steps to protect those victims from serious abuse and neglect.

The Intellectual Disability (Compulsory Care and Rehabilitation) Act 2003 provides for a compulsory care and rehabilitation programme for individuals with intellectual disabilities. Compulsory care orders can be made by the court if these individuals have been found unfit to stand trial for an offence resulting in imprisonment. In addition, the Criminal Procedure (Mentally Impaired Persons) Act 2003 allows the court to proceed with further investigation of a defendant's mental status, and to order that a person be detained as a special patient in hospital instead of sentencing him or her to imprisonment.

Policies and Programmes

According to the Ministry of Health (n.d.), mental health is a priority health area for the New Zealand government as mental illness accounts for a significant proportion of the total burden on health care resources. To mitigate the burden of mental health, several important initiatives have been implemented to provide support and treatment for people with mental illness, and at the same time, promote mental health in older people.

The 2001 New Zealand Positive Ageing Strategy is the main initiative directing social services and programmes for older New Zealanders. The primary aim of this strategy is to provide a framework for developing social policy for older people, through monitoring and reviewing the actions of central and local government authorities across the nation (Ministry of Social Development 2001). This strategy consists of 10 goals which guide policies and programmes to improve opportunities for older people to participate in their communities in ways they choose. The strategy's focus on 'positive' ageing and participation emphasises the promotion of mental health from a more holistic orientation that goes beyond simply offering treatment for mental illnesses or disorders among older people.

The 2002 Health of Older People Strategy is particularly pertinent to mental health care for older people in New Zealand. The strategy aims to provide a framework for developing an integrated approach to health and disability support services for older people (Ministry of Health 2002). The main focus of this strategy is on improving health care programmes and promotion actions and is mainly conducted by the Ministry of Health and local DHBs. The strategy also seeks to ensure that service providers work closely with an older person's whānau, carers, and communities, and that rapport is established at all times.

Specifically in the mental health area, the Ministry of Health has focused on a recovery approach to mental illness since the late 1990s. The main principle of this approach is underpinned by the belief that mental health and wellbeing is about living well in the presence or absence of a mental disorder. The emphasis of this approach lies in assisting recovery for service users and promoting their mental health and wellbeing. Based on this approach, the government's five-year strategy (Rising to the Challenge: The Mental Health and Addiction Service Development Plan 2012–2017) has been implemented to ensure that people with mental health and addiction issues have better access to care and services in the community (Ministry of Health 2012). This plan includes specific actions to be delivered by the Ministry of Health, DHBs and mental health and addiction service providers to improve the health and wellbeing of people with mental illness and addiction issues.

Another government initiative in the mental health area is the Like Minds, Like Mine project, initiated by the Ministry of Health in 1997. The main aim of this public education programme is to reduce the stigma of mental illness, as well as preventing and/or tackling discrimination against people with mental illness in the community (Ministry of Health, n.d.). According to the project website, this is "one of the first comprehensive national campaigns in the world to counter stigma and discrimination associated with mental illness" (Like Minds, Like Mine, n.d., n.p.). Through this nationwide project, national television campaigns and stigma watch activities have taken place to improve attitudes and behaviour of individuals and groups towards those people experiencing mental illness. A cost-benefit analysis of this programme showed that the public's attitudes towards people with mental illness have improved significantly since the programme was established in 1997 (Vaithianathan, cited in Ministry of Health and Health Promotion Agency 2014).

Aligned with the New Zealand Positive Ageing Strategy and the de-stigmatising campaigns of Like Minds, Like Mine, the Mental Health Foundation has recently launched a website and wellbeing project focused on the maintenance of wellbeing amongst older New Zealanders (www.boomers.org.nz). Using personal narratives and modelled on 'saving for retirement' models of fiscal planning, the project emphasises successful mental health ageing as a process of connection, engagement and participation.

Mental Health Practice

Mental health needs of older adults are mainly channelled through the primary general health providers represented by general medical practices. Primary health care addressed through primary health organisations (PHOs), which are centred on general practitioner (GP) surgeries, where community-based support, assessment and treatment will occur. This approach provides the opportunity for partnerships with specialist providers in non-governmental organisations, and for referral to secondary and tertiary services such as Mental Health Services for Older People, located within DHBs, whose prime focus is assessment and treatment for age-related dementias, depression and other mental health disorders occurring as a result of ageing. For those older people with a pre-existing mental health disorder prior to their reaching the age of 65, it is assumed that they will continue to receive service from an adult mental health team. Limited acute in-patient facilities exist for older people, with most mental health concerns being addressed within community settings, either in a person's own home or in rest home facilities.

The Ministry of Health (2011) estimates that some 60% of residents in rest home settings experience some level of dementia: most rest homes are run by charities or by the commercial sector, with funding for individual care being means-tested and underpinned by state welfare provision. Some care facilities have dedicated dementia units, but there is often a familiar practice issue involving the determination of suitability, transition of people between residential facilities as their mental state deteriorates, and the engagement and involvement of families in care decisions.

NGO practice involvement with older people with mental health concerns is widespread but under-resourced. For older people and their families, it is often hard to navigate across the range of providers to locate available services. For those living in isolation, through geographical, income-related or sensory isolation, access to services is not universally available and the risk of depression is therefore heightened. Isolation from families, through urbanization, colonization and migration, emerges as a major practice issue.

CURRENT ISSUES AND CHALLENGES

Under-detection and limited resourcing for the problem of elder abuse remain of concern. The majority of elder abuse teams are located within Age Concern New Zealand (NGO), which also provides visiting, housing and budgeting services aimed at supporting wellness in ageing. Other significant NGOs provide support for those living with, or caring for, those with Alzheimer's and other dementias, and those experiencing the effects of strokes, Parkinson's, and other diseases.

The growing ethnic diversity in New Zealand's cities presents a practice challenge, with Auckland (New Zealand's largest city, with over 1.42 million people) rapidly becoming one of the world's most multicultural cities, particularly in terms of Asian migrants and their descendants. Arguably, generational transitions from cultures where expectations of 'filial piety' (Sung 2007) are the norm, to communities where familial obligation and welfare are more individualized and less generationally interdependent, create a growing demand for culturally specific and sensitive practice delivery.

On a positive note, mental health practice with older people has embraced a recovery perspective, with primary health strategies focused on positive ageing and a recognition that effective mental health intervention is often achieved by community-level, holistic processes and organisations. One example is the Men's Shed movement (www.menzshed.org.nz), which has a focus on practical 'handyman' (sic) projects and community engagement that provide companionship and the opportunities for health education. Targeted health promotion campaigns such as rural mental health and men's initiatives are aimed at creating capacity for resilience in future generations of older people.

The majority of mental health services that older people receive are provided by social service professionals, although many of these practitioners are not trained specifically in mental health or specifically in the management of aged care. Specific topics like dementia alone require specific training to enable social service professionals to have in-depth knowledge for intervention and informed support. However, mental health is also an area that is closely tied to the updates in medical knowledge and research. This necessitates not only a need for specialized training, but continuous professional development.

In supporting older people with mental health issues, there is a need to consider that there may be other, coexisting, medical conditions alongside prescribed medications that further complicate and challenge the situation. It is critical that issues of mental health be addressed and included in health and ageing policies as mental disorders have a direct impact on physical health (Knight and Sayegh 2011). Carer stress (physical, emotional, social and financial) is a crucial issue, as is the need to respond to the stereotyping on ageing and mental health (Karlin and Fuller 2007).

Conclusion

In order to improve the services and care of older adults with mental health needs, there is a need to move beyond a single model of intervention and instead facilitate multiple systems of care. The New Zealand scenario for older people is one that is made up of both settler populations and indigenous Māori. Each cultural community brings their own informed model of care and intricate sensitivities. In line with social work practice from an ecological perspective, a client-centred approach in collaboration with all relevant stakeholders is not only sensitive, but more likely to contribute to effective and long-term successful intervention. New Zealand's demographic profile is rapidly changing: the numbers of older people will have doubled by the year 2050, and this group will be significantly more ethnically and culturally diverse. Generational changes in attitudes to older people, changes in family size and definition, continuing urbanisation and its impact on housing, are all factors that will have a bearing on the mental health needs of older people. The rise in incidence of depression as a result of social isolation and financial hardship is a trend that requires urgent policy attention.

There is considerable need for new approaches to economic planning, health care and welfare support, retirement policies, alongside innovative living space arrangements, engaging inter-generational relations and management of more constructive views on ageing.

Acknowledgments

The authors express great appreciation to Aram Kim, Senior Psychiatric Registrar at Waitemata District Health Board, and Erin Loo, University of Canterbury, for their comments and suggestions.

REFERENCES

Abbott, M. W., Wong, S., Williams, M., Au, M. K., and Young, W. (1999). Chinese migrants' mental health and adjustment to life in New Zealand. *Australian and New Zealand Journal of Psychiatry*, 33, 13–21.

Broadstock, M., Brinson, D., and Weston, A. (2008). The effectiveness of compulsory, residential treatment of chronic alcohol or drug addiction in non-offenders: A systematic review of the literature. Christchurch, New Zealand: Health Services Assessment Collaboration (HSAC), University of Canterbury.

Budge, C., Stephens, C., and Stichbury, C. (2014). Health: Summary report for the New Zealand longitudinal study of ageing. Palmerston North, New Zealand: Massey University.

Chapman, D. P., Perry, G. S., and Strine, T. W. (2005). The vital link between chronic disease and depressive disorders. *Preventing Chronic Disease,* 2(1), 1–10.

Dulin, P. L., Stephens, C., Alpass, F., Hill, R. D., and Stevenson, B. (2011). The impact of socio-contextual, physical and lifestyle variables on measures of physical and psychological wellbeing among Māori and non-Māori: The New Zealand health, work and retirement study. *Ageing and Society,* 31(08), 1406–1424.

Durie, M. (1998). Whaiora: Maōri health development (2nd ed.). Auckland, New Zealand: Oxford University Press.

Gray, A., and Elliott, S. (2001). Refugee resettlement research project: 'Refugee voices': Literature review. Wellington, New Zealand: New Zealand Immigration Service.

Harvey, S. (2013, August 26). Elderly suicide rate higher than others. Stuff. Retrieved from http://www.stuff.co.nz/national/9088438/Elderly-suicide-rate-higher-than-others.

Ho, E., Au, S., Bedford, C., and Cooper, J. (2003). Mental health issues for Asians in New Zealand: A literature review. Wellington, New Zealand: Mental Health Commission.

Ikin, J. F., Creamer, M. C., Sim, M. R., and Mckenzie, D. P. (2010). Comorbidity of PTSD and depression in Korean War veterans: Prevalence, predictors, and impairment. *Journal of Affective Disorders,* 125(1–3), 279–286.

Karlin, B. E., and Fuller, J. D. (2007). Meeting the mental health needs of older adults. *Geriatrics,* 62, 26–35.

Khan, N., Davis, P., Wilkinson, T. J., Sellman, J. D., and Graham, P. (2002). Drinking patterns among older people in the community: Hidden from medical attention? *New Zealand Medical Journal*, 115, 72–75.

Khan, N., Wilkinson, T. J., and Keeling, S. (2006). Reasons for changing alcohol use among older people in New Zealand. *Australasian Journal on Ageing,* 25(2), 97–100.

Knight, R. G., and Sayegh, P. (2011). Mental health and aging in the 21st century, *Journal of Aging and Social Policy*, 23(3), 228–243.

Kuruvilla, G., Davidson, T., McCabe, M., Mellor, D., and Moore, K. (2007). Treatment of depression in low-level care residential facilities for the elderly. *International Psychogeriatrics*, 19(6), 1153–1160.

Laracy, K., Trimmer, W., and Love-Gray, M. (2011). Mental health in primary care: A resource for New Zealand health professionals. Porirua, New Zealand: Whitireia New Zealand.

Like Minds, Like Mine. (n.d.). About. Retrieved from http://www.likeminds.org.nz.

Long, N., Macdonald, C., and Chamberlain, K. (1996). Prevalence of posttraumatic stress disorder, depression and anxiety in a community sample of New Zealand Vietnam War veterans. *The Australian and New Zealand Journal of Psychiatry,* 30(2), 253–256.

Ministry of Health. (n.d.). Mental health. Wellington, New Zealand: Author. Retrieved from http://www.health.govt.nz/our-work/mental-health-and-addictions/mental-health.

Ministry of Health. (2002). Health of Older People Strategy. Wellington, New Zealand: Author.

Ministry of Health. (2011). Mental health and addiction services for older people and dementia services: Guideline for district health boards on an integrated approach to mental health and addiction services for older people and dementia services for people of any age. Wellington, New Zealand: Author.

Ministry of Health. (2012). Rising to the challenge: The mental health and addiction service development plan 2012–2017. Wellington, New Zealand: Author.

Ministry of Health and Health Promotion Agency. (2014). Like minds, like mine national plan 2014–2019: Programme to increase social inclusion and reduce stigma and discrimination for people with experience of mental illness. Wellington, New Zealand: Author.

Ministry of Social Development. (2001). New Zealand positive ageing strategy. Wellington, New Zealand: Author.

Oakley Browne, M. A., Wells, J. E., and Scott, K. M. (2006). Te rau hinengaro: The New Zealand mental health survey. Wellington, New Zealand: Ministry of Health.

OECD. (2013). Pensions at a glance 2013: OECD and G20 indicators. Paris, France: OECD Publishing.

Park, H. (2014). Living with 'Hwa-byung': The psycho-social impact of elder mistreatment on the health and well-being of older people. *Aging and Mental Health,* 18(1), 125–128.

Perkins, C. (2013). Dementia, what you need to know: A guide for people with dementia, and their caregivers. Auckland, New Zealand: Random House New Zealand.

Perry, B. (2010). The material wellbeing of older New Zealanders. Background papers of the Retirement Commissioner's 2010 review. Wellington, New Zealand: Ministry of Social Development.

Polotu-Endemann, F. K. (2009). Fonofale model of health. Retrieved from http://www.hauora.co.nz/resources/Fonofalemodelexplanation.pdf.

Statistics New Zealand. (2006). Demographic aspects of New Zealand's ageing population. Retrieved from http://www.stats.govt.nz/browse_for_stats/people_and_communities.

Statistics New Zealand. (2014a). 2013 Census ethnic group profiles. Retrieved from http://www.stats.govt.nz/browse_for_stats/snapshots-of-nz.

Statistics New Zealand. (2014b). New Zealand in profile: 2014. Retrieved from http://www.stats.govt.nz/browse_for_stats/snapshots-of-nz/nz-in-profile-2014.aspx.

Stephens, C., Alpass, F., and Towers, A. (2010). Economic hardship among older people in New Zealand: The effects of low living standards on social support, loneliness, and mental health. *New Zealand Journal of Psychology,* 39(2), 49–56.

Sung, K.-T. (2007). Respect and care for the elderly: The East Asian way. Lanham, MD: University Press of America.

In: Ageing and Mental Health: Global Perspectives
Editors: Wendy Wen Li, Sherry M. Cummings et al.
ISBN: 978-1-63484-777-3

Chapter 6

AGEING AND MENTAL HEALTH: CHALLENGES AND INNOVATIONS IN HONG KONG

Alma Au[1, *], Ho-ming Yip[1], Wai-chi Chan[2], Xue Bai[1] and Teresa Tsien[1]

[1]Hong Kong Polytechnic University, Hung Hom, Hong Kong
[2]The University of Hong Kong, Pokfulam, Hong Kong

ABSTRACT

Like many cities and countries around the world, Hong Kong is facing challenges posed by an ageing population. Subsequently, there is a greater pressure on services and caregivers to provide appropriate and sufficient care to the elderly, especially those suffering mental illness. This chapter aims to examine the socio-cultural context that shapes Hong Kong's service orientation of mental illness for older adults, and to review mental health services for older adults and caregivers. Through highlighting the challenges related to service development and population ageing as well as the recent initiatives of the Hong Kong Government, we hope to highlight possible directions in translational research, and provide recommendations for the future development of mental health services for the elderly.

Keywords: active ageing, caregiving, stigma, volunteering, strength-based, community support

INTRODUCTION

Hong Kong is facing challenges posed by an ageing population. According to the Hong Kong Population Projections 2012-2041, the percentage of the population aged 65 and over is projected to rise markedly from 13% in 2011 to 30% in 2041 (Census and Statistics Department of the Government of the Hong Kong Special Administration Region, 2012).

* Corresponding author: Alma Au, Hong Kong Polytechnic University. Email: alma.au@polyu.edu.hk.

Ageing population is a result of two primary determinants: a fall in fertility rates and a rise in life expectancy. The increasing ageing population in Hong Kong would pose more challenges to mental health services in addressing the needs of older adults and their caregivers. This chapter aims to reveal the socio-cultural context that shapes Hong Kong's service orientation of mental illness for older adults, mental health services for older adults with mental illness and caregivers with a view to identifying the possible recommendations for enhancing mental health services in Hong Kong.

Context of Ageing and Mental Health in Hong Kong

Culture is thought to have an impact on how a society perceives ageing and mental health, the stigma attached to mental illness, and the coping strategies employed by those with mental health problems. The Hong Kong Chinese culture of valuing an older person as a 'treasure at home' has been eroding and replaced with negative stereotypes of older people as frail, dependent, and non-productive. This shifting perception is further reinforced by a decline in the social status of older adults as a result of low education and the lack of retirement pensions (Cheng, Chan and Chan, 2008). The culture of ageism affects the mental health of older adults. Bai, Lai and Guo (In press) have observed that there was a positive correlation between depression in older adults and age-related stereotypes that consider older adults as a burden and besieged with mental health problems. Through long-term exposure to these negative stereotypes, older adults tended to internalise these negative images leading to a sense of inadequacy, low self-esteem and depression (Bai and Chow, 2011; Rodin and Langer, 1980).

In addition to ageism, public stigma against patients with mental illness in Hong Kong further leads to discrimination of older adults with mental illness and their caregivers. Public stigma refers collectively to the unwarranted stereotype, prejudice, and discriminatory practices against a social group that are widely shared by members of a society because they possess attributes that are considered undesirable, disgraceful, or objectionable (Rusch, Angermeyer and Corrigan, 2005). The prevalence of public stigma to mental illness is due to the lack of public understanding about the nature of the illness. Studies have indicated that those with a psychiatric condition are considered 'weird' or 'crazy' and different from the 'normal people' (Tsang, Tam, Chan and Cheung, 2003). Such stigma is associated with distress and depression in patients and caregivers (Mak et al., 2007; Perlick et al., 2007). Moreover, the public stigma on mental illness affects the provision of mental health service to older adults with mental illness, and discourages patients from continuing treatment (Sirey et al., 2001). Such stigma also has an impact on the establishment of service centres supporting those with mental illness. For example, expansion of Integrated Community Centres for Mental Wellness ("ICCMWs") in all eighteen districts in Hong Kong is made difficult mainly as a result of opposition by local residents and community leaders (Equal Opportunities Commission, 2014).

Issues concerning social stigma and 'face saving' are prevalent in Chinese cultures. Having a family member diagnosed with mental illness is considered shameful and family members feel guilty as it is seen as tarnishing the family honour, name, and ancestors (Ng, 1997). Concealment and denial are often used to help family members cope with the stigma. For example, it is common for persons with dementia not to seek medical attention until the symptoms have persisted for long periods of time and the illness is at an advanced stage (Chow et al., 2002; Sheng, Law and Yeung, 2009). As a result, the stigma creates social exclusion that prevents older adults with mental illness from maintaining involvement in the community.

In view of the negative stereotypes on ageing and mental illness, it is important to commit to transforming public perceptions and ideas about these concepts. The government, healthcare professionals, older adults themselves, as well as the rest of the society to overcome such prejudice and discrimination; to recognise older adults' strengths and contributions; to enable them to age in place with dignity; and to let them share their wisdom and voice their needs (Minichiello, Browne and Kendig, 2000). To achieve this, a Policy Framework (WHO, 2002) to promote the concept of "active ageing" was formulated. Active ageing was defined as "the process of optimising opportunities for health, participation and security in order to enhance quality of life as people age," and allows "people to realise their potential for physical, social, and mental well-being throughout the life course and to participate in society…, while providing them with adequate protection, security and care when they require assistance" (p. 12). This framework shifts the focus on perceiving older adults as unproductive and frail to one of 'productivity' and 'generativity' as core elements of positive ageing.

A positive attitude to ageing has also been associated with better physical and mental health, and life satisfaction (Bryant et al., 2012). Enhancing social cohesion, social participation, community engagement, and physical activity leads to a significant improvement in physical and mental health and quality of life of older adults, as well as improving the quality of community life (Au, Lai and Ng., 2015; Au and Tsien, 2013; Taylor et al., 2004). As such, these are important facets for preventing or delaying disease and various forms of disabilities associated with old age. There is growing interest in developing and evaluating structured intervention programmes to promote productive and active ageing. These programmes emphasise investment in the future by enhancing coping competencies in middle and late adulthood (Bode et al., 2007). The Hong Kong government has stepped up effort in promoting a culture of active ageing as a way to facilitate the elderly and support them in leading a more fulfilled life in their golden years. This is done through harnessing their wealth of experience, knowledge, and expertise through continued learning, volunteer service, and participation in social and economic activities. Various centres such as the Neighbourhood Elderly Centre (NEC) and the District Elderly Community Centre (DECC) organise educational, social and recreational activities for elders. Similarly, the Labour and Welfare Bureau (LWB) and the Elderly Commission have also collaboratively organised a variety of projects and activities such as the Neighbourhood Active Ageing Project, the Elder Academy Scheme, and the production of radio programmes.

Prevalence of Mental Health Problems in Hong Kong

Previous local studies have suggested that dementia (Chiu et al., 1998; Lam et al., 2008; Lam et al., 2010; Wu et al., 2014; Yu et al., 2012), depression (Chan et al., 2006; Chan et al., 2012; Chi et al., 2005) and suicide (Chiu et al., 1996; Ho, 2003; Yip, 1996; Yip et al., 2003) are common issues associated with mental health problems among older adults in Hong Kong.

Dementia

Dementia is a common mental health issue among older adults. There has been an increasing prevalence rate of dementia in Hong Kong since 1995. A local community study with a sample of 6,100 older Chinese people in Hong Kong estimated that 9.3% of adults aged 70 and above (women: 15.3%; men: 8.9%) had clinically diagnosed dementia in 2005 (Lam et al., 2008). In comparison, another study involving 1,034 older adults from the community reported that 6.1% of participants had been diagnosed with dementia (Chiu et al., 1998). A study by Yu et al. (2012) that applies the prevalence rate of previous studies (Census and Statistics Department of Hong Kong Special Administrative Region, 2001; 2005; 2009; Chiu et al., 1998; Lam et al., 2008) projected that the number of people aged 60 and above with dementia would increase from 103,433 in 2009, to 332,688 in 2039.

Dementia becomes more prevalent with increasing age (Chiu et al., 1998; Lam et al., 2008; Yu et al., 2012). A study by Chiu et al. (1998) indicated that the incidence of dementia approximately doubles for every 5 years. By the age of 90, approximately one in four older persons would have developed dementia.

Compared to older adults living in the community, older adults living in institutions tend to have a higher prevalence rate of dementia. The Census and Statistics Department of Hong Kong Special Administrative Region (2009) showed that 31.6% of institutional elderly aged 60 or above are reported to have dementia. This can be related to situations in which dementia is often associated with compromised self-care abilities.

Depression

Depression is a common mental illness among the elderly. A local community study with 917 Chinese adults in Hong Kong showed that the prevalence of depression among those aged 60 or above was 11% and 14.5% for men and women respectively (Chi et al., 2005). The prevalence of depression tends to increase with their age. Chou and Chi's (2005) community study with 1,903 older people in Hong Kong found that the prevalence rate was greater for the oldest old (aged 80 and above: 31.1%) than the old-old (aged between 70 and 79: 22.4%) and young-old (aged between 60 and 69: 19.1%). Studies have suggested that older adults living in an institution have a higher prevalence of depression than those living in the community (Chow et al., 2004; Seitz, Purandare and Conn, 2010). For instance, a local study with 245 samples of private nursing home residents revealed a prevalence rate of depression was 29% for older people aged 65 or above (Chow et al., 2004).

Suicide

Suicide risk in Hong Kong tends to increase across the life course for both men and women, with the highest suicide rates occurring among the oldest age groups (Yip, 1996). According the Hospital Authority (2011), the overall suicide rate of older adults aged 65 or above was 26.4 per 100,000, which was much higher than the overall suicide rate of 15.2 per 100,000 in Hong Kong in 2006. Regarding suicide ideation, a study by Yip et al. (2003) using a sample of 917 older people in Hong Kong aged 60 or above reported that 5.5% of elderly people expressed a wish to commit suicide.

Mental Health Services for the Elderly

At present, there is no elderly mental health policy in Hong Kong. The service direction follows the principle of 'ageing in place as the core, and institutional care as back-up'. Community-based services are provided by non-governmental organisations and the Hospital Authority[1] to support older adults with mental illness and assist them in remaining part of the community for as long as possible. Mental health services for older adults are delivered through an integrated service delivery model that covers prevention, early identification, medical treatment and rehabilitation services provided within the community (Hospital Authority, 2012). This means older adults with serious mental illness will be supported by inpatient and residential care. These services are provided in multi-disciplinary and cross-sectoral settings through the collaboration and cooperation of the Hospital Authority, the LWB, Social Welfare Department (SWD), Department of Health, non-governmental organisations, and other stakeholders in the community.

The overall responsibility for coordinating the various mental health service programmes is assumed by the Food and Health Bureau. In the light of the growing ageing population their growing mental health needs, the Food and Health Bureau created the Review Committee on Mental Health in May 2013. This Committee comprised members such as legislative councillors, academics, healthcare professionals, service providers, service users and caregivers, as well as representatives from the Equal Opportunities Commission and the Hong Kong Council of Social Services. A subgroup has also been created to study the service needs of elders and make recommendations for mental health services and relevant policy measures (Legislative Council Panel on Health Service, 2014).

The existing mental health services for older adults are subsumed under both medical and social service systems. The medical system consists of primary, specialist services and hospital care for rehabilitation. The social service system covers community support services and residential care services.

Mental Health Services under the Medical System

Primary Care

Primary care for mental health services provides accessible, first contact care that is comprehensive, continuing, co-ordinated, and person-centred in the context of family and community (Food and Health Bureau, 2010). These services are mainly provided by the Hospital Authority and the Department of Health. A number of services on early intervention, medical treatment, and community support services are provided to improve care and support for mental health patients in the community. Since the 1990s, the Department of Health has systematically launched various programmes as preventive measures to promote mental health in later life. The General Out-patient Clinic (GOPC) service is a community-based primary care service to provide medical treatment to older adults with mental illness. Efforts have also been made to extend the scope of the primary care system through closer collaboration among primary care providers, specialists, and social service sectors. For

[1] The Hospital Authority manages all public hospitals in Hong Kong. It is governed and monitored by the Secretary for Food and Health.

example, an Integrated Mental Health Program (IMHP) for patients with common mental disorders is covered in all clusters to engage more patients with the primary care services. Patients under the care of Hospital Authority with stabilised and milder mental health conditions would also be referred to GOPCs for further management by family medicine specialists and general practitioners working in multi-disciplinary teams (Food and Health Bureau, 2012).

Specialist Psychiatric Service

Specialist psychiatric service is the secondary level of care that is meant to be curative in nature. It is mainly provided by medical specialists either in the community or a hospital setting. Specialist psychiatric services in the community include Specialist Out-patient Clinics (SOPC) and Community Psychogeriatric Teams. Psychiatry Specialist Out-patient Clinics are located in different districts to provide psychiatric services to patients in the community. Former mentally ill persons, including older adults, are entitled to receive follow-up consultations at SOPC upon their return to the community. Some of the specialist out-patient clinics, such as Kwai Chung - Psychogeriatric Out-patient Department cum Carers Support Centre, are specifically to serve the psychiatric needs of older adults.

Meanwhile, the Hospital Authority delivers community psychiatric outreach services to older adults with mental illness through its Community Psychogeriatric teams in Pamela Youde Nethersole Eastern Hospital, Queen Mary Hospital, Kowloon Hospital, United Christian Hospital, Yung Fung Shee Memorial Centre, Castle Peak Hospital, Kwai Chung Hospital, North District Hospital, and Shatin Hospital. Among the services provided by the Community Psychogeriatric teams are designated care, rehabilitation programmes, home visits to elders with mental illness aged 65 or above, a memory clinic, the Elderly Suicide Prevention Program (ESPP), and the Enhanced Home and Community Care Scheme (EHCCS). Others are Nurse-led Outreach Services to selected, subsidised Old Age Homes (OAHs) and Nursing Homes, Psychogeriatric Nurse Clinics (PGNC), Mobile Cognitive Assessment Clinics (MCAC), Dementia Supplement (DS) Verification Exercises, home visits by multi-disciplinary members, and educational and training programmes.

The psychogeriatric outreach teams also provide consultation to elders in residential care homes for older adults (RCHEs) with varying degrees of mental health problems such as dementia and depression. This service currently covers around 110 subsidised residential care homes for the elderly and over 200 private establishments all over Hong Kong. A total of 73,513 psychogeriatric outreach attendances were recorded in 2013 (Legislative Council Panel on Health Service, 2014). As for elders with a chronic mental disorder, inpatient care in hospital is provided. Being in hospital care means older adults can have access to extended care that caters to their complex needs that require a longer period of rehabilitation in the hospital. These rehabilitation activities include life-skills training, social group interaction, orientation programmes, physical training, multi-sensory stimulation, and reminiscence therapy.

Mental Health Services under Social Service System

Community Support Services

Community support services are provided to facilitate older adults with mental illness to re-integrate into the community. To strengthen and integrate the community-based support for mentally ill patients, including older adults, the Social Welfare Department has initiated the Integrated Community Centre for Mental Wellness (ICCMW) in all districts across the territory since October 2010. Through the integrated service mode, the ICCMW provides one-stop, district-based, accessible community support and social rehabilitation services. These services, provided from a single entry point, ranged from early prevention to risk management for discharged mental patients, persons with suspected mental health problems, their families and carers, and residents living in the serving district. Apart from outreach services and casework counselling services, the scope of ICCMW's services also include therapeutic and support group service, social and recreational activities, day training, occupational therapy training services for outreach, and public education programmes on mental health that tailor to the unique needs of older adults with different levels of mental illness. The effect of the community-based support services, however, is limited by the stigmatisation of mental illness in the community. The opposition from the local residents and community leaders creates barrier for some ICCMWs to locate permanent service sites (Equal Opportunities Commission, 2014).

As for the needs of older adults with different levels of dementia, several subvented and non-subvented elderly centres, including the Neighbourhood Elderly Centre (NEC), District Elderly Community Centre (DECC), and Day Care Centre, provide community support services. These centres support older individuals to remain in the community and also to provide support for family caregivers who are unable to care for patients during the day. Different elderly centres offer different levels of community support services depending on the dementia patients' level of impairment. For example, day care centres provide services during daytime to dementia elders of moderate to severe level of impairment. Apart from personal and nursing care services, rehabilitation and social and recreational services are provided to dementia elders to help them maintain an optimal level of functioning and improve their quality of life.

Residential Care Services

While older adults are encouraged to live in the community, older adults who have a severe cognitive impairment or mental illness may have difficulty remaining in the community if their caregivers are unable to look after them. Therefore, mentally ill older adults who have a low level of self-care ability are supported by residential care. For them, the Social Welfare Department provides various residential care services. Long stay care homes (LSCH) are long-term residential care and active maintenance services for chronic mentally ill patients. Regarding older adults with dementia, residential care services are provided by both non-governmental organisations and private sectors. Residential care provided by non-governmental organisations includes both subsidised and non-subsidised homes for the aged, care and attention homes, and nursing homes.

Mental Health Policies Related to Older People

Apart from aforementioned mental health services provided in medical and social welfare settings, there are also legal protections for older adults with mental illness including the provision of guardianship and financial management. The Mental Health Ordinance 136 covers provision for guardianship to mentally incapacitated persons. Under Section 59J, a body corporate called the Guardianship Board was established to provide guardianship for adults aged 18 years and over with a mental disorder. Upon the provision of a guardianship order, the appointed guardian can manage the personal affairs, financial matters, or medical or dental treatment of the mentally incapacitated person. Meanwhile, the Enduring Powers of Attorney Ordinance (Cap. 501 of the Laws of Hong Kong) allows an individual to choose the person or persons who will look after his/her financial affairs in the event that he/she becomes mentally incapacitated.

Informal Caregiving in Hong Kong

Compared to mental health services provided to older adults, support for family caregivers has received little attention in Hong Kong (Tsien and Ng, 2010). In line with the service direction of ageing in place, family members become the major caregivers supporting older adults with mental health problems to remain in the community. The prevalence of family caregivers taking care of older adults with mental illness has undergone significant changes due to the evolving socio-economic situation in Hong Kong. The rise of the nuclear family and the increase in female employment make adult children or daughters-in-law less likely to take care of older adults (Chong, Kwan, Chi, Lou and Leung, 2014). In light of this and the reduced likelihood of cohabitating with children, spouses are increasingly stepping into the role of caregivers (Sugiura, Ito, Kutsumi and Mikami, 2009). A local study revealed that spousal caregivers represented 26.3% of all family caregivers in Hong Kong in 2009 (Chow and Ho, 2012).

Social support can enhance well-being and self-efficacy of Chinese caregivers (Au et al., 2009a). In particular, the emotional support provided by family members was found to have a significant correlation with enhanced life satisfaction and decreased depressive symptoms in the caregivers (Au et al., 2009b). Nonetheless, many caregivers often become secluded for prolonged periods in the course of adopting the caregiving role, where the possibility of seeking social support through face-to-face contacts becomes diminished. Moreover, in the context of maintaining relational harmony and avoiding social sanctions, Chinese caregivers have reported concerns about others' evaluation and expectations of themselves as well as losing face and avoiding both direct confrontations and disclosures of personal difficulties even within the family itself (Au, Shardlow, Teng, Tsien and Chan, 2013).

Being the caregiver of an older person with a mental disorder on a daily basis provides significant demands and challenges. Among different types of mental disorders experienced by older adults, caregivers for older adults with dementia have attracted much attention both in China and Hong Kong. Local research suggested that the burden of caring for a family member with dementia is associated with deteriorated physical health, reduced psychological well-being and increased risk of depressive mood (Ho, Chan, Woo and Sham, 2009). Discontinuity of the social network occurs when family caregivers have to take up the daily caring responsibility that results in decrease in social participation and loss of emotional support. Local studies have also revealed that confusion over dementia diagnosis, the difficulties in handling dementia patients' behavioural problems, and a lack of coping methods to handle the illness present significant challenges to families and caregivers, and these challenges need to be addressed (Chan et al., 2010). To relieve caregiving stress, there is an increasing trend of family members employing domestic helpers to assist in the caregiving role (Asato, 2004; Bai, Kwok, Chan and Ho, 2013). Domestic helpers reduce caregivers' roles by providing personal care support to a care-recipient including dressing, hygiene, mobility, toileting needs, escorting them to outdoor activities and attending medical consultation. However, the use of domestic helpers to reduce caregivers' stress is debatable. Domestic helpers might not be effective as caregivers for dementia patients due to a lack of specific training, communication difficulties and the need to address other domestic duties.

To facilitate family members to care for older adults with mental illness in the community, community-based support services are provided to support caregivers in social service settings (Chong et al., 2014). Psycho-educational support, case counselling, and mutual support groups are provided to caregivers of mentally ill older adults through the ICCMW, and to caregivers of older adults with dementia through the NEC, District Elderly Community Centre (DECC), and day care centres. However, these community-based support services might not be adequate in meeting the needs of family caregivers. First of all, the aforementioned community-based non-governmental organisations are centre-based and operate on weekdays with a nine-to-five working schedule. The constraints in a centre-based service with limited working hours may prevent caregivers from seeking face to face meetings with counsellors due to caregiving duties. Moreover, the nature of these services is mainly focused on psychosocial support while the practical needs of caregivers, such as manageing challenges in caregiving duties, assistance with attendance at medical consultations and financial difficulties, might not be met.

THE WAY FORWARD: BUILDING HUMAN CAPITAL

According to the Hong Kong Population Projections 2012-2041, the percentage of the population aged 65 and over is expected to rise markedly from 13% in 2011 to 30% in 2041 (Census and Statistics Department of the Government of the Hong Kong Special Administration Region, 2012). Many of these people are working or have had work experience. Like many other well-developed countries, Hong Kong is not spared the challenges of an ageing population. The proportion of the population aged 65 and over is projected to rise markedly from just over 900,000 or 13% of the population in 2011 to over 2.5 million or 30% of the population in 2041. Nearly one third of Hong Kong's population will be aged 65 or above in 2041, while the retirement age is 60. The population census carried out by the Census and Statistics Department of the Hong Kong Special Administrative Region (2011) also indicated declining labour force participation. This is attributable to the continual increase in share of oldest old amongst all older persons. The median monthly income from main employment of the working older persons in 2011 was HK$8500 (approximately US$1094 in 2011), which is 77.3% of the median income (HK$11,000) of the entire working population. The low median income of older adults can be related to the low wages of the occupations they were engaged in which in turn were determined by their relatively low educational attainment. Financial problems have been found to be a significant risk factor of suicidal ideation among older adults in Hong Kong (Yip et al., 2003).

The Legislative Council Commission of Hong Kong Special Administrative Region (2014) has made various recommendations for preparations for population ageing and the shrinking work force in Hong Kong. These recommendations have implications on how mental health services for older adults are going to evolve. Measures include encouraging more people to work beyond their usual retirement age through measures to recruit and retain mature workers, promoting work-life balance for female populations, and helping caregivers to balance work and care responsibilities. Furthermore, to enable active ageing and productivity, investment in human capital has to be made through life-long learning and employment-related training. At the same time, innovations such as the use of assisted living technology and interventions supported by the internet or telephone are being promoted to support the elderly and their family members. Finally, in the light of the increasing trend of employing domestic helpers to take up caregiving duties in Hong Kong, health care and government officials would need to consider providing domestic helpers with relevant training in dementia care and management (Chong et al., 2014).

The active old in Hong Kong are often very keen to learn new skills and to contribute to society through participation in volunteer work and paid employment (Au and Tsien, 2013). In addition to achieving productive ageing, another local study strongly supports the notion that community-based volunteer support is an effective method to support the needs of caregivers (Au et al., 2015; Au, Lai and Ng, 2015). This community-based volunteer support program was designed to test a model designed for intervention with dementia caregivers through telephone support, consisting of both psychoeducational and behavioural activation (BA) practice components, to reduce the burden of caregivers. The project examined the feasibility and effectiveness of some of the components to be delivered by telephone to increase accessibility and sustainability for caregivers. Results suggested that competence-based training could be effectively administered through telephone with the help of senior citizens volunteering as paraprofessionals. Sustainable social support to caregivers is important to their mental health (Au et al., 2009a). The findings of the above study on telephone-assisted support for caregivers have long-term implications. First of all, the study suggests that young old could be a source of volunteer support that relieves caregivers' burden and stress. Second, the nature of telephone support can be an alternative mode of community support to provide services to caregivers who do not have time for face-to-face services (Au et al., 2015).

Benefits associated with volunteering among senior citizens are well-documented. These include reduced symptoms of depression, better self-reported health, fewer functional limitations and lower mortality (Musick and Wilson, 2003). There is also evidence to suggest that volunteering for pro-social reasons and that feeling one's effort matters are associated with greater benefits (Anderson et al., 2014; Au, Ng, Gardner, Lai and Chan, 2015; Morrow-Howell et al., 2003). There are also very specific programmes offered in ageing-friendly communities in which older adults act as peer counsellors to fellow older adults to promote positive ageing (Gonzales and Morrow-Howell, 2009).

The erosion of Hong Kong Chinese culture of valuing an older person as a treasure at home and the filial piety model of care (Cheng, Chan and Chan, 2008) can have major implications for the mental health of older adults. Considering Hong Kong has high standards of living, the long-term erosion of care together with sustained exposure to the negative stereotypes of older adults can create extreme challenges for older adults and even worse for people with dementia and mental illness. Promoting a strength-based approach to mental health management for older adults can be further encouraged through capitalising on community resources in the provision of sustainable mental health services (Au, Ng, Gardner, Lai and Chan, 2015; Cheng, Lau, Mak, Ng and Lam, 2014; Tsien and Ng, 2010).

REFERENCES

Anderson, N. D., Damianakis, T., Kroger, E., Wagner, L. M., Dawson, D. R., Binns, M. A., ... BRAVO Team (2014). The Benefits Associated with Volunteering among Seniors: A Critical Review and Recommendations for Future Research. *Psychology and Ageing, 140*, 1505-1533.

Au, A., Gallagher-Thompson, D., Wong, M. K., Leung, J., Chan, W., Chan, C.C, Lu, H. J., Lai, M. K. and Chan, K. (2015). Behavioral activation for dementia caregivers: scheduling pleasant events and enhancing communications. *Clinical Interventions in Ageing, 10*, 611-619.

Au, A., Lai, M. K., Lau, K. M., Pan, P. C., Lam, L., Thompson, L. and Gallagher-Thompson, D. (2009a). Social support and well-being in dementia family caregivers: The mediating role of self-efficacy. *Ageing and Mental Health, 13*(5), 761-768.

Au, A., Lai, S. and Ng, E. (2015). Forward to Special Issue: Positive Ageing in Action. In A. Au. and D. Gallagher-Thompson (Eds.) Special Issue on Working with Older Adults: Innovations and Implementations. *Clinical Gerontologist, 38* (3), 187-189.

Au, A., Lau, K. M., Koo, S., Cheung, G., Pan, P.C. and Wong, M. K. (2009b) The Effects of Informal Social Support on Depressive Symptoms and Life Satisfaction in Dementia Caregivers in Hong Kong. *Hong Kong Journal of Psychiatry, 19*, 57-64.

Au, A., Li, S., Lee, K., Leung, P., Pan, P.-C., Thompson, L. and Gallagher-Thompson, D. (2010). The Coping With Caregiving group program for Chinese caregivers of patients with Alzheimer's disease in Hong Kong. *Patient Education and Counseling, 78*(2), 256-260.

Au, A., Ng, E., Gardner, B., Lai, S. and Chan, K. (2015). Proactive Ageing and Intergenerational Mentoring Program to Promote the Well-being of Older Adults: Pilot Studies. In A. Au. and D. Gallagher-Thompson (Eds.) Special Issue on Working with Older Adults: Innovations and Implementations. *Clinical Gerontologist, 38* (3), 203-210.

Au, A., Shardlow, S. M., Teng, Y., Tsien, T. and Chan, C. (2013). Coping strategies and social support-seeking behaviour among Chinese caring for older people with dementia. *Ageing and Society, 33*(8), 1422-1441.

Au, A. and Tsien, T. (2015). *Goals and successful ageing.* Invited Presentation as Outstanding Paper for 20th Annual Congress of Gerontology organized by the Hong Kong Association of Gerontology.

Bai, X. and Chow, N. (2011). How is the self-image formed and enhanced among older Chinese people: through assimilation or contrast? *Asian Journal of Gerontology and Geriatrics, 6*(1), 22-28.

Bai, X., Lai, D. W. L. and Guo, A. (in press). Ageism and depression: Perceptions of older people as a burden in China. *Journal of Social Issues*, *72*(1).

Bai, X., Kwok, T. C., Chan, N. Y. and Ho, F. K. (2013). Determinants of job satisfaction in foreign domestic helpers caring for people with dementia in Hong Kong. *Health and Social Care in the Community*, *21*(5), 472-479.

Bode, C., de Ridder, D. T., Kuijer, R. G. and Bensing, J. M. (2007). Effects of an intervention promoting proactive coping competencies in middle and late adulthood. *The Gerontologist*, *47*(1), 42-51.

Bryant, C., Bei, B., Gilson, K., Komiti, A., Jackson, H. and Judd, F. (2012). The relationship between attitudes to ageing and physical and mental health in older adults. *International Psychogeriatrics*, *24*(10), 1674-1683.

Census and Statistics Department of Hong Kong Special Administrative Region. (2001). *Special Topics Report No. 27.* Retrieved from http://www.statistics.gov.hk/pub/B11301272001XXXXB010.pdf.

Census and Statistics Department of Hong Kong Special Administrative Region. (2005). *Thematic Household Survey Report No. 21.* Retrieved from http://www.statistics.gov.hk/pub/B113022120-05XXXXB0100.pdf.

Census and Statistics Department of Hong Kong Special Administrative Region. (2009). *Thematic Household Survey Report No. 40.* Retrieved from http://www.statistics.gov.hk/pub/B113024020-09XXXXB0100.pdf.

Census and Statistics Department of Hong Kong Special Administrative Region. (2012). H*ong Kong Population Projection 2012-2041.* Retrieved from http://www.statistics.gov.hk/pub/B1120015052012XXXXB0100. pdf.

Census and Statistics Department of Hong Kong Special Administrative Region. (2013). *2011 Population Census Thematic Report: Older Persons.* Retrieved from http://www.statistics.

Chan, D., Kwok, A., Leung, J., Yuen, K., Choy, D. and Leung, P. C. (2012). Association between life events and change in depressive symptoms in Hong Kong Chinese elderly. *Journal of affective disorders*, *136*(3), 963-970.

Chan, S. W., Chiu, H. F., Chien, W. T., Thompson, D. R. and Lam, L. (2006). Quality of life in Chinese elderly people with depression. *International Journal of Geriatric Psychiatry*, *21*(4), 312-318.

Chan, W., Ng, C., Mok, C., Wong, F., Pang, S. and Chiu, H. (2010). Lived experience of caregivers of persons with dementia in Hong Kong: A qualitative study. *East Asian Archives of Psychiatry*, *20*(4), 163-168.

Cheng, S. T., Chan, W. and Chan, A. (2008). Older people's realisation of generativity in a changing society: the case of Hong Kong. *Ageing and Society*, *28*(5), 609-627.

Cheng, S. T., Lam, L. C. and Kwok, T. (2013). Neuropsychiatric symptom clusters of Alzheimer disease in Hong Kong Chinese: Correlates with caregiver burden and depression. *The American Journal of Geriatric Psychiatry*, *21*(10), 1029-1037.

Cheng, S., Lau, R., Mak, E., Ng, N. and Lam, L. (2014). Benefit-finding intervention for Alzheimer caregivers: Conceptual framework, implementation issues, and preliminary efficacy. *The Gerontologist*, *54*(6), 1049-1058.

Chi, I., Yip, P. S., Chiu, H. F., Chou, K. L., Chan, K. S., Kwan, C. W., . . . Caine, E. (2005). Prevalence of depression and its correlates in Hong Kong's Chinese older adults. *The American Journal of Geriatric Psychiatry*, *13*(5), 409-416.

Chiu, H., Lam, L., Chi, I., Leung, T., Li, S., Law, W., . . . Lum, C. (1998). Prevalence of dementia in Chinese elderly in Hong Kong. *Neurology*, *50*(4), 1002-1009.

Chiu, H. F., Lam, L. C., Pang, A. H., Leung, C. and Wong, C. (1996). Attempted suicide by Chinese elderly in Hong Kong. *General hospital psychiatry*, *18*(6), 444-447.

Chong, A., Kwan, C., Chi, I., Lou, V. and Leung, A. (2014). Domestic helpers as moderators of spousal caregiver distress. *The journals of gerontology. Series B, Psychological sciences and social sciences*, *69*(6), 966-972.

Chou, K. L. and Chi, I. (2005). Prevalence and correlates of depression in Chinese oldest-old. *International Journal of Geriatric Psychiatry*, *20*(1), 41-50.

Chow, E. O. and Ho, H. C. (2012). The relationship between psychological resources, social resources, and depression: Results from older spousal caregivers in Hong Kong. *Ageing and mental health*, *16*(8), 1016-1027.

Chow, L., Siu, E., Hei Kong, B. M., Wong, P., Tak, M., Draper, B., . . . Wong, C. (2004). The prevalence of depressive symptoms among elderly Chinese private nursing home residents in Hong Kong. *International Journal of Geriatric Psychiatry*, *19*(8), 734-740.

Chow, T., Liu, C., Fuh, J., Leung, V., Tai, C., Chen, L. W., . . . Chen, Q. (2002). Neuropsychiatric symptoms of Alzheimer's disease differ in Chinese and American patients. *International Journal of Geriatric Psychiatry*, *17*(1), 22-28.

Equal Opportunities Commission of Hong Kong. (2014). *Mental Health Policy and Services Submission from the Equal Opportunities Comission*. Retrieved from http://www.legco.gov.hk/yr13-14/english/panels/hs/papers/hs0616cb2-1788-2-e.pdf.

Food and Health Bureau of the Hong Kong Special Administrative Region. (2010). *Primary care development in Hong Kong strategy document*. Retrieved from http://www.fhb.gov.hk/download/press_and_publications/otherinfo/101231_primary_care/e_strategy_doc.pdf.

Food and Health Bureau of the Hong Kong Special Administrative Region. (2012). *Hong Kong Reference Framework for Preventive Care for Older Adults in Primary Care Settings*. Retrieved from http://www.pco.gov.hk/english/resource/files/ref_framework_adults.

Food and Health Bureau of the Hong Kong Special Administrative Region. (2014). Review on Mental Health – Strengthening Mental Health Services for Adults. Retrieved from http://www.legco.gov.hk/yr13-14/english/panels/hs/papers/hs0428cb2-1340-3-e.pdf.

Ho, S. C., Chan, A., Woo, J., Chong, P. and Sham, A. (2009). Impact of Caregiving on Health and Quality of Life: A Comparative Population-Based Study of Caregivers for Elderly Persons and Noncaregivers. *The Journals of Gerontology. Series A, Biological Sciences and Medical Sciences*, *64*(8), 873-879.

Ho, T. P. (2003). Psychiatric care of suicides in Hong Kong. *Journal of affective disorders*, *76*(1), 137-142.

Hospital Authority of Hong Kong. (2011). *Mental health service plan for adults 2010-2015*. Retrieved from http://www.ha.org.hk/upload/publication_42/372.pdf.

Hospital Authority of Hong Kong. (2012). *Strategic service framework for elderly patients*. Retrieved from http://www.ha.org.hk/upload/publication_42/369.pdf.

Lam, L. C., Lee, J. S., Chung, J. C., Lau, A., Woo, J. and Kwok, T. C. (2010). A randomized controlled trial to examine the effectiveness of case management model for community dwelling older persons with mild dementia in Hong Kong. *International Journal of Geriatric Psychiatry*, *25*(4), 395-402.

Lam, L. C., Tam, C. W., Lui, V. W., Chan, W., Chan, S. S., Wong, S., . . . Chan, W. (2008). Prevalence of very mild and mild dementia in community-dwelling older Chinese people in Hong Kong. *International Psychogeriatrics*, *20*(01), 135-148.

The Legislative Council Commission of Hong Kong Special Administrative Region. (2014). *Preparing for population ageing*. Retrieved from http://www.legco.gov.hk/research-publications/english/1415rb01-preparing-for-population-ageing-20141113-e.pdf.

Mak, W. W., Cheung, R. Y., Law, R. W., Woo, J., Li, P. C. and Chung, R. W. (2007). Examining attribution model of self-stigma on social support and psychological well-being among people with HIV+/AIDS. *Social Science and Medicine*, *64*(8), 1549-1559.

Minichiello, V., Browne, J. and Kendig, H. (2000). Perceptions and consequences of ageism: views of older people. *Ageing and Society*, *20*(03), 253-278.

Morrow-Howell, N., Hinterlong, J., Rozario, P. A. and Tang, F. (2003). Effects of volunteering on the well-being of older adults. *The Journals of Gerontology Series B: Psychological Sciences and Social Sciences*, *58*(3), S137-S145.

Morrow-Howell, N., Hong, S. I. and Tang, F. (2009). Who benefits from volunteering? Variations in perceived benefits. *The Gerontologist*, gnp007.

Musick, M. A. and Wilson, J. (2003). Volunteering and depression: The role of psychological and social resources in different age groups. *Social Science and Medicine*, *56*(2), 259-269.

Ng, C. H. (1997). The stigma of mental illness in Asian cultures. *Australian and New Zealand Journal of Psychiatry*, *31*(3), 382-390.

Perlick, D. A., Miklowitz, D. J., Link, B. G., Struening, E., Kaczynski, R., Gonzalez, J., . . . Rosenheck, R. A. (2007). Perceived stigma and depression among caregivers of patients with bipolar disorder. *The British Journal of Psychiatry*, *190*(6), 535-536.

Rüsch, N., Angermeyer, M. C. and Corrigan, P. W. (2005). Mental illness stigma: concepts, consequences, and initiatives to reduce stigma. *European psychiatry*, *20*(8), 529-539.

Rodin, J. and Langer, E. (1980). Ageing labels: The decline of control and the fall of self-esteem. *Journal of Social Issues*, *36*(2), 12-29.

Seitz, D., Purandare, N. and Conn, D. (2010). Prevalence of psychiatric disorders among older adults in long-term care homes: a systematic review. *International Psychogeriatrics*, *22*(07), 1025-1039.

Sheng, B., Law, C. B. and Yeung, K. M. (2009). Characteristics and diagnostic profile of patients seeking dementia care in a memory clinic in Hong Kong. *International Psychogeriatrics*, *21*(02), 392-400.

Sirey, J. A., Bruce, M. L., Alexopoulos, G. S., Perlick, D. A., Raue, P., Friedman, S. J. and Meyers, B. S. (2001). Perceived stigma as a predictor of treatment discontinuation in young and older outpatients with depression. *American Journal of Psychiatry*, *158*(3), 479-481.

Sugiura, K., Ito, M., Kutsumi, M. and Mikami, H. (2009). Gender differences in spousal caregiving in Japan. *The Journals of Gerontology. Series B, Psychological Sciences and Social Sciences*, *64*(1), 147-156.

Taylor, A., Cable, N., Faulkner, G., Hillsdon, M., Narici, M. and Van Der Bij, A. (2004). Physical activity and older adults: a review of health benefits and the effectiveness of interventions. *Journal of Sports Sciences*, *22*(8), 703-725.

Tsang, H. W., Tam, P. K., Chan, F. and Cheung, W. (2003). Stigmatizing attitudes towards individuals with mental illness in Hong Kong: Implications for their recovery. *Journal of Community Psychology*, *31*(4), 383-396.

Tsien, T. B. and Ng, G. T. (2010). Older adults as caregivers in Hong Kong. *China Journal of Social Work*, *3*(2-3), 231-245.

United Nations, Department of Economic and Social Affairs, Population Division. (2013). *World Population Ageing 2013*. Retrieved from http://www.un.org/en/development/desa/population/publications/pdf/ageing/WorldPopulationAgeing2013.pdf.

World Health Organization. (2002). *Active ageing: A policy framework*. Retrieved from http://whqlibdoc.who.int/hq/2002/WHO.

Wu, Y. T., Lee, H. Y., Norton, S., Prina, A. M., Fleming, J., Matthews, F. E. and Brayne, C. (2014). Period, birth cohort and prevalence of dementia in mainland China, Hong Kong and Taiwan: a meta-analysis. *International Journal of Geriatric Psychiatry*, *29*(12), 1212-1220.

Yip, P. (1996). Suicides in Hong Kong, Taiwan and Beijing. *The British Journal of Psychiatry*, *169*(4), 495-500.

Yip, P. S. F., Chi, I., Chiu, H., Chi Wai, K., Conwell, Y. and Caine, E. (2003). A prevalence study of suicide ideation among older adults in Hong Kong SAR. *International Journal of Geriatric Psychiatry*, *18*(11), 1056-1062.

Yu, H., Chau, P., McGhee, S., Cheung, W., Chan, K., Cheung, S. and Woo, J. (2012). Trends in prevalence and mortality of dementia in elderly Hong Kong population: projections, disease burden, and implications for long term care. *International Journal of Alzheimer's Disease*, *2012*, 1-6.

In: Ageing and Mental Health: Global Perspectives
Editors: Wendy Wen Li, Sherry M. Cummings et al.
ISBN: 978-1-63484-777-3

Chapter 7

AGEING AND MENTAL HEALTH IN SOUTH KOREA

***Dongbae Kim*[1,*] *and Hyo Jung Lee*[2]**
[1]Yonsei University, Seoul, South Korea
[2]University of Massachusetts, Boston, MA, US

ABSTRACT

The current health care system in South Korea puts less emphasis on mental health concerns and their treatments compared to physical illnesses, because Koreans tend to be reluctant to discuss their mental health issues or seek help. Korea is now experiencing the fastest expansion in the world in terms of the proportion of older adults among its population. With this rapid increase in the older population, meeting the various needs of this age group, especially regarding mental health, has become one of the major policy issues in Korea. This is in response to the growing prevalence of dementia and depression, increasing incidents of abuse and neglect against older adults, and the highest suicide rates of the elderly among the Organization for Economic Cooperation and Development (OECD) countries. In the past, caregiving of older adults was provided mainly by family members, particularly women, and it was considered a virtue of the adult children. But in recent years, due to the unprecedented increase in the number of frail elderly, the Korean government has developed policies and services to help these older citizens and their families: the National Long-term Care Insurance, the Elderly Care Services, the Dementia Management Act, and others. This chapter provides an overview of older Koreans' mental health issues by examining multiple aspects: the cultural and contextual aspect, epidemiology of mental disorders in older adults, mental health-related social services and policies, and caregiving issues. Gaps in current policy, practice, and research are also discussed.

Keywords: caregiving, mental health, mental health services and policies, older Koreans

* Corresponding author: Dongbae Kim, Yonsei University. Email: eagle207@yonsei.ac.kr.

INTRODUCTION

South Korea (hereafter, Korea) has experienced huge demographic changes over the past 20 years. These changes include a rapid increase in the number of older adults, a fast growth in the proportion of older adults among the population, and a significant drop in the fertility rate (Statistics Korea, 2011). In 2012, 11.8% of Koreans were older than 65 (Korean Statistical Information Service [KOSIS], 2014). One of the most striking features of ageing in Korea is the rapid expansion in the proportion of older adults: it will take only 18 years for the share of Korea's population aged 65 or older to increase from 7% (in 2000) to 14% (projected in 2018) (Statistics Korea, 2011). The same transition took longer for other developed countries in OECD, such as Japan (26 years, from 1970 to 1996), United Kingdom (45 years, from 1930 to 1975), the United States (69 years, from 1944 to 2013), and France (115 years, from 1865 to 1980) (Kinsella and He, 2009; OECD, 2013).

This unprecedented growth of the older population in Korea has a direct impact on the increasing needs of this age group. The financial security and maintenance of good health are priorities for this group and their family members. Compared to physical health issues, however, mental health issues and psychological well-being of senior citizens in Korea have not been fully addressed yet (Ko et al., 2012). Therefore, in this chapter, we aim to provide an overview of ageing and mental health issues in Korea from multiple aspects. We commence with the culture and context of ageing in Korean society and then focus on the prevalence of several key mental health disorders in senior Koreans. We also discuss mental health services available for older Koreans. We then continue with caregiving issues in Korea and mental health related policies for older adults and families, followed by a description of the gaps in policy, practice, and research in the field of ageing and mental health in Korea. The concluding section will suggest some implications for future studies in the field of ageing and mental health in Korea.

MENTAL HEALTH IN OLD AGE: KOREAN CULTURE AND CONTEXT

According to Korean tradition, reaching old age has been perceived as a blessing on a personal level, since very few people reached their late years (Choi, 2009; Sung, 2001). In the Korean context, older persons, especially older men, are described as people with wisdom, as leaders, and as counselors of family and community. However, this positive perception of being older has altered with modernisation of society and the unprecedented ageing process (Choi, 2009; Sung, 2001). In recent years, many older adults have been characterised by negative features such as being financially dependent or in a state of poverty (about 45% of older adults live in poverty), socially isolated, and physically vulnerable (Jung et al. 2012; Kim and Cook, 2011). These negative stereotypes attached to older Koreans tend to exacerbate health issues. For instance, some older adults who experience age discrimination devalue or marginalise themselves due to ageism, which may contribute to or be associated with poorer psychological, physical, and social well-being in late life.

Research indicates that mental health in late life is an area which has somehow been neglected (Ko et al., 2012). One reason for this could be culturally initiated: Koreans are more likely to perceive psychological concerns as a personal weakness or a lack of determination

(Cho, Lee, Kim, Lee and Sohn, 2011). Therefore, in general, Koreans are reluctant to disclose their mental health issues or to seek help (Kim et al., 2011; Seoul National University Hospital, 2011). It may also be related to the fact that difficulties in mood or mind sometimes present similarly to physical symptoms that Asian older adults frequently report (Shin and Lukens, 2002). The other reason mental health issues are overlooked could be the implicitly pervasive thought that these concerns are not considered health conditions (Cho et al., 2011). Some older persons may think their rapid memory decline or depressive symptoms are part of normal ageing. Therefore, detecting mental health difficulties, much less treating them, in older Koreans is a challenge.

Prevalence of Older Koreans' Mental Health Disorders

The most commonly discussed mental health disorders in the older population are dementia and depression (Oh et al., 2014). Older Koreans have reported that dementia is the most feared disease, followed by stroke and cancer (Cho et al., 2011; Jung et al., 2012; Seoul National University Hospital, 2009).

Dementia

The most recent epidemiologic studies in Korea show that 8.1% to 8.7% of older adults aged 65 and over are suffering from some type of dementia (Cho et al., 2011; Kim et al., 2011; Kim et al., 2014). This percentage is somewhat similar to those of other developed countries such as the United States, Canada, the United Kingdom, and Italy (6.6%~13.9%), and greater than those of other Asian countries such as Japan (4.8%~7.2%) and China (1.8%~4.0%) (Seoul National University Hospital, 2009; Kim and Han, 2012; Kim et al., 2014). Alzheimer's disease is the most prevalent type of dementia (5.7%) in older Koreans followed by vascular dementia (2.0%) (Kim et al., 2011). Epidemiologic studies indicate that the key risk factors for dementia among Korean elders are: advanced age, being female, lower education attainment level (or illiteracy, common in this age group in Korea), smoking, history of head trauma, and depression (Cho et al., 2011; Kim et al., 2010).

Depression

Depression in late life has attracted scholars' and policy makers' attention because Korea has had the highest suicide rate among the OECD countries for years, and depression is indicated as one of the major reasons of suicide especially in late life. Now, the public has begun to recognise the importance of mood and its impact on overall well-being (Jeon, 2011; Cho et al., 2011). According to a nationally representative epidemiologic study that surveyed older adults between 65 and 74, the life-time prevalence of major depressive disorder (MDD) is 6.4% (of older people in the survey) while the life-time prevalence of dysthymia is 1.2%. The one-year prevalence of MDD is 2.8% to 3.0% while that of dysthymia is 0.7% to 0.8%. These results were found by using fully-structured interviews like the Composite International Diagnostic Interview (CIDI) (Cho et al., 2011). When using semi-structured interviews, however, 5.4% to 9.4% of older adults were identified as having MDD (Cho and Sohn, 2013; Cho et al., 2011; Lee, Choi, Jung and Kwak, 2000; Park et al., 2010). Compared to all other age groups, except for adults aged 18 to 29 whose one-year prevalence is 4.0%, the one-year prevalence of depression among senior citizens aged 70 and older is the highest in Korea (3.8%) (Seoul National University Hospital, 2011). This prevalence rate is distinctive from other countries that show a decreased prevalence of depression in people with advanced age. Studies indicate that risk factors for depression in older Koreans include advanced age and being female, illiterate, cognitively impaired, and chronically ill (Cho and Sohn, 2013; Cho et al., 2011; Kim et al., 2014).

Anxiety

Anxiety disorders are common mental health concerns in childhood and throughout adulthood (Kessler, Chiu, Demler, Merikangas and Walters, 2005). However, compared to western countries including the United States (18.1%) and France (12.0%), Korean adults (aged 18 to 64) show a relatively lower one-year prevalence of anxiety disorders (6.8%) (Cho et al., 2011). In older Koreans (aged 60 to 74), the one-year prevalence of anxiety disorders is 5.7% (Cho et al., 2011). Research from other countries indicates that in early to late adulthood, women are more likely than men to be diagnosed with anxiety disorders (McLean, Asnaani, Litz and Hofmann, 2011). This is true in Korea, too. A higher one-year incidence rate of anxiety is found in adult women (9.8%) compared to their male counterparts (3.7%) (Seoul National University Hospital, 2011). Women aged 60 and older show the lowest one-year incidence risk of anxiety (6.7%~8.8%) compared to women in younger age groups (aged 18 to 59; 8.1% to 12.6%). To the contrary, men aged 70 to 74 show the highest one-year incidence risk of anxiety (4.4%) of all male age groups (2.5% to 3.8%), except for young men aged 18 to 29 (5.2%).

Aside from these major mental health disorders, a few other conditions have recently been brought to the public's awareness regarding older Koreans' well-being such as sleep disorders, substance abuse, and delirium (Cho and Sohn, 2013; Cho et al., 2011; Kim et al., 2012).

In general, older Koreans at risk of mental health disorders or problems often show similar patterns of social difficulties such as living alone, residing in rural areas or having low income (Seoul National University Hospital, 2009; Oh, 2013), all of which are attracting the attention of researchers and policy makers to this demographic. Such difficulties are strongly associated with mental health problems in later life either as a cause or an effect: sometimes these difficulties trigger or facilitate mental health problems; meanwhile, mental health problems influence older persons' socio-economic, physical and emotional troubles. The following sub-section will briefly describe two mental health related issues among older Koreans, 1) elder abuse and neglect and 2) later-life suicide, which seem to be phenomena of a deadlock of the cause and/or effect.

Mental Health Related Issues in Late Life

One of significant mental health related issues related to older Koreans is elder abuse and neglect. These problems are related to older people's low levels of self-esteem, relatively low social status, and lack of social roles in the modernised and individualised Korean society. According to the 2009 National Elder Abuse Incidence Study and the National Survey of Senior Citizen in 2011, approximately 13% of Korean elders experienced physical, psychological, or other types of abuse and neglect (Korea Institute for Health and Social

Affairs [KIHASA], 2010; Jung et al., 2012; Jung, 2013). The most frequently reported type of abuse was psychological (emotional) abuse (67%), followed by neglect (22%) (KIHASA, 2010). These victims are more likely to be female, single, and older (KIHASA, 2010). They also tend to live in rural area, to have lower socioeconomic status, to have poorer health, and to be socially isolated (KIHASA, 2010). The vast majority (71.9%) of the abusers are the older victims' own children and children in-law. Only 2.5% of these victims seek formal help from outside (e.g., police, local elderly protection agency), while about two-thirds (65.7%) do nothing. These victims show lower levels of self-esteem, feel depressed, and blame themselves for the abuse (KIHASA, 2010; Jung et al., 2012).

Another critical mental health related phenomenon in older population is the high suicide rate. In Korea, the suicide rate for all ages was 29.8 per 100,000 in 2012, which is far higher than the average rate of the OECD countries (13.2 per 100,000) (OECD, 2013). In particular, out of 100,000 older Koreans, 42.4 in their 60's, 73.1 in their 70's, and 104.5 in their 80's committed suicide in 2012: these were the highest among the OECD countries (KOSIS, 2014; OECD, 2013). These numbers are also far higher than those of any other age groups in Korea - 19.5 out of 100,000 people in their 20's, 27.3 in their 30's, 30.9 in their 40's, and 35.3 in their 50's (KOSIS, 2014). These numbers indicate that older Koreans may be more at risk of suicide than any other age group in Korea and any other OECD countries. One of the most common causes for elderly suicide in Korea is mental or psychiatric problems (including depression, loneliness) along with physical illnesses, financial problems, and family conflicts (Chang, 2012; Statistical Research Institute, 2007).

Mental Health Services for Older Koreans

Korea has developed mental health services and programs to address the rising concern for mental health issues such as dementia, depression, and anxiety which are associated with abuse, neglect, and high suicide rate in older adults. In general, older Koreans' health care expenses (including mental health care expenses) are covered by the National Health Insurance, a universal social insurance program for all Koreans. For those with financial disadvantage, the National Medical Aid Program covers their health costs. In 2008, the National Long-term Care Insurance (LTC), a universal social insurance program, was implemented. In addition, private insurance plans are available to provide further coverage to fill the gap for people who can afford such insurance or choose to purchase it for the supplementary coverage.

More than three decades after the initial mental health policy was established in 1960, the new Mental Health Act was passed in 1995. It stressed Social Restoration Services (ambulatory psychosocial rehabilitation services in the community) to reduce long-term hospitalisation and to invigorate the community-based mental health services. Currently, Korea has a community-based mental health service delivery system that consists of 18 national and/or public mental hospitals, 200 community mental health centers, and 255 community rehabilitation centers along with 1,270 private mental health hospitals and clinics (Ministry of Health and Welfare (MOHW), 2014). Community mental health centers are operated under the guidance of the public health centers and university-affiliated hospitals. These centers provide counselling, home visits, case-management, educational activities and programs, and vocational rehabilitation. Community rehabilitation centers are mainly focused on rehabilitating patients with mental health disorders to help them make a smooth transition back into the community. The centers offer therapeutic work programs, vocational rehabilitation, individual and group therapy, and transitional living programs.

As a response to the high suicide rate which is the fourth highest cause of death in Korea, the Suicide Prevention Law was enacted in 2011 and then implemented in 2012. Under this law, the National Suicide Prevention Center and local Suicide Prevention Centers were established. These centers provide counselling services, public education, and emergency hotlines to help people at risk. In addition, a national call center aimed at suicide prevention is operated by the Ministry of Health and Welfare (Korea Suicide Prevention Center, 2014). Note that these centers provide services accessible to people of all ages. However, in response to the high suicide rate in older Koreans, suicide prevention and intervention programs specially targeting older adults have been designed and developed.

In addition, the Dementia Management Act (DMA) established mental health care services targeting older people and their family members. As a result of the growing number of older adults with dementia and the expansion of individual, familial, and social costs of this disease, the DMA was legislated in 2011 and has been functioning since 2012. This act provides governmental involvement to support older patients and their family members by building national and local dementia management centers. In 2014, there were a total of 256 dementia management centers and 830 professionals working in these centers (National Assembly Budget Office, 2014). The DMA also provides legal support to deliver counseling and daycare services at local community health centers. In order to identify dementia patients in the early stages of the disease, a dementia screening test for community-dwelling older adults is provided by these centers. From 2008 to 2011, about a half of older Koreans (46%) received the dementia screening test and 2.5% of these persons were diagnosed with dementia (National Assembly Budget Office, 2014).

CAREGIVING FOR OLDER ADULTS IN KOREA

Needs for care in late life are often assessed based on current health conditions, disability levels, or chronic or acute diseases of older individuals. Research on caregiving and caregivers of older adults in Korea is mostly linked to functional limitations in daily living or to the specific health conditions of care recipients. For instance, approximately 15% of older Koreans experience at least one limitation in Activities of Daily Living (ADLs)[1] or Instrumental Activities of Daily Living (IADLs)[2] (Jung et al., 2012). Among older adults with at least one functional limitation, only 23.6% report that they receive informal and/or formal care. Among older adults receiving some types of care, 72.1% report that family members are their primary source of care, 13.1% receive care from both family members and outside services, and 11.4% receive care only from outside the home. These percentages confirm that older adults with functional limitations rely heavily on family members to receive some types

[1] Seven items of ADLs were included: 1) dressing, 2) personal hygiene, 3) bathing, 4) eating, 5) walking, 6) toileting, and 7) experiencing incontinence.

[2] Ten items of IADLs were included: 1) glooming, 2) doing housework, 3) preparing meals, 4) doing laundry, 5) taking medications, 6) managing money, 7) going out within the community, 8) shopping, 9) using telephone, and 10) handling transportation.

of care. However, more than three quarters of older adults with functional limitations still receive no care at all. The elderly care insurance pilot study evaluation report (KIHASA, 2006) presents similar findings (N = 5,368). Even though 9.9% of respondents demonstrated depression, 7.7% suffered from insomnia, 3.4% reported hallucinations, and 16% to 20% of respondents experienced difficulties in several cognitive activities, only 35.3% of respondents reported that they had caregivers while 64.7% had none.

Informal caregivers are mostly family members of older adults in Korea. According to research, caregivers of older adults aged 65 to 74 are mostly 60 years and older, whereas those giving care to older adults aged 80 years and older are relatively younger, being 40 to 60 years old (Jung et al., 2012; KIHASA, 2006). These findings reflect the demographic tendency that older adults in the relatively lower age category are more likely to be married and their main caregivers are spouses who themselves are also older adults, while older adults in the relatively higher age category are more likely to be bereaved or single and have poorer health. This suggests that these age groups are more likely to be taken care of by their children or spouses of children. By far, women are more likely to take the role as a primary caregiver than are men, regardless of age. In Korea, the first son and daughter-in-law's role is still significant in caregiving. In particular, the daughter-in-law often becomes a primary caregiver providing hands-on care such as preparing food, dressing, and bathing, whereas her spouse (son of care recipient(s)) is more likely to provide financial support to parents. In the majority of cases, the daughter-in-law provides care for her parents-in-law due to marital obligation and not because of voluntary fondness for these parents-in-laws; this often produces a greater caregiving burden for the daughter-in-law during the caregiving period (Knight et al., 2002; Lee, Yoon and Kropf, 2007).

Regarding mental health issues in later life, caregiving for older adults with dementia has attracted much public attention. In 2009, the Nationwide Study on the Prevalence of Dementia in Korean Elders interviewed caregivers of older adults with dementia. Among these caregivers, 68.5% were women with an average age of 60.8 years. More than 40% of caregivers in this study were spouses of the patient, 16.7% were daughters-in-law, 15.3% were daughters, and 15.3% were sons. Sixty five percent of these caregivers either lived with the patient or met with the older patient every day. More than 60% of them did not work for pay. These caregivers' average number of caregiving hours per week was 33.6; this is much greater than the average caregiving hours of caregivers of older adults with functional limitations in ADLs and IADLs (20.3 hours per week) (KIHASA, 2006). Although more than seven out of ten caregivers report caregiving as a burden (including psychological, physical, and financial aspects), more than one-third of these caregivers report that they have never thought about institutionalising these older care recipients (e.g., in a nursing home, geriatric hospital). However, it is also evidenced that these caregivers are more likely to be depressed, to have lower levels of well-being, and to have more physical or health problems (Seoul National University Hospital, 2009).

As shown earlier, caregiving for older adults has heavily relied on assistance from family members in Korea. Based on cultural norms in Korea, the Confucian virtue of filial piety (e.g., respect for older parents), the phenomenon of adult children living with their parents and providing informal care for them has been considered normal (Chee and Levkoff, 2001; Knight et al., 2002; Lee, Yoon and Kropf, 2007). However, there have also been demographic and social changes that affect these traditional beliefs concerning caregiving in Korean society. These shifts include the rapidly growing number of older adults, the significant decrease in the number of older adults co-residing with their adult children, the considerable increase in the number of women working outside of the home, and evolving cultural norms as a mixture of traditional and modern or market principles (Goldsmith, 2012; Jones, 2010).

A recent nationwide survey reflects these changes (Jung et al., 2012). For instance, a 2011 survey found that 68.1% of older adults lived alone or lived only with spouses, compared to 40.4% in 1994 and 55.0% in 2004 (Jung et al., 2012). In addition, seven out of ten older Koreans reported that as they get older they prefer to live by themselves, not with their adult children. This survey also showed that older Koreans prefer to be financially independent (85.6%); only 14.2% of them considered relying on their children to obtain financial sources to live. Given all these statistics, there has been an increasing need for formal care for older Koreans. As a response to this need, the Korean government has introduced the LTC insurance and has enhanced home- and community-based services for older adults to provide sufficient care and support for them and their caregivers.

Mental Health Related Policies for Older Adults and Their Families

In Korea, there are three components of the social welfare system: 1) social insurance (health insurance, national pension, worker's compensation, unemployment relief, and long-term care), 2) public assistance (livelihood protection, medical aid, veterans relief, disaster relief), and 3) social welfare services (for people with physical and/or mental disability, older adults, children, and women). Across these three components, there are policies and services to support older adults and their families and to promote their well-being. This section introduces these policies and services with a focus on two separate groups: older adults and their family members.

First is the National Long-term Care Insurance (LTC), a universal program active since 2008. The LTC aims to promote quality of life among older adults and their families and to mitigate the negative impact of geriatric illnesses and disabilities on individual, familial, and social outcomes by sharing the burden at the societal level. The LTC provides both health care and welfare services through two channels: residential care and home-based services with both in-kind and cash benefits (but cash benefits are only for those living in rural areas with no adequate service facility). Residential care includes nursing homes (about 30 to 300 residents) and share houses (5 to 9 residents, e.g., the Green House homes in the U.S.). In 2013, the number of nursing homes supported and supervised by the government was 1,501 and 3,084 were operated by individuals, for a total of 4,585 residential care homes. Meanwhile, home-based services for community-dwelling older adults include home-help, home-visit bathing, home-visit nursing, day care, short-term stay, and appliance rental.

Those aged 65 years and over who have functional limitations in daily living, regardless of types of illnesses, are eligible for the LTC services. In 2013, 378,000 or 6.1% of all older Koreans received LTC (Statistics Korea, 2013). People younger than 65 years old are also eligible when their functional limitations are caused by selected geriatric illnesses such as dementia, stroke, and Parkinson's disease. There is no means test for eligibility for the LTC; however, functional limitation levels are comprehensively, somewhat strictly, evaluated by assessors (mostly nurses and social workers in government agencies) dispatched by the

National Health Insurance Services. In 2013, 41.3% of LTC expenditures were given to recipients with dementia, and the increased rate of expenditure to this group (recipients with dementia) is much higher (18.8% per year) than that of LTC recipients in general (8.7% per year) (National Assembly Budget Office, 2014).

Initially, the LTC beneficiaries are classified into three care levels depending on their degree of disability. The LTC beneficiaries with the first and second care levels receive the institutional benefits while only paying for out-of-pocket cost (which is 20% of the total cost). Those beneficiaries with the third care level benefit from home-based services and they are only liable for 15% of the total cost as out-of-pocket. Beneficiaries of livelihood protection are exempt from any payment. In 2014, the LTC policy of classification of care levels was amended to meet complex needs of older Koreans and their family members. As of July 1, 2014, the previous three care levels were expanded to include a fourth care level, and a special fifth care level was also created to actively respond to service needs of older adults with dementia and cognitive dysfunctions and those of their family members.

Second, within the Social Security Act, there is the Community Care Service for the elderly. This Community Care Service contains three service components: preventive services, building of social security net services, and emergency services. Preventive services are daily life activity support, emotional support, home modification, leisure, counselling, and community resource development. The building of social security nets includes educational support, community network building, and service coordinating and linking. Emergency services comprise abuse or neglect assessment, short-term stays in a shelter, and emergency alert system. Local community welfare centers or senior welfare centers are a base to deliver services such as delivery of meals, haircuts, shaving, counselling, educational programs, or emergency intervention services. Those eligible to obtain these services include older adults who have no care or support from a legal guardian or caregiver (normally, spouses or adult children) or ones who receive public assistance (e.g., livelihood protection recipients). Generally, low-income older adults with functional limitations who are not eligible for the LTC are qualified for all these community care services.

Third, the Elderly Care Comprehensive Service, started in 2007, is one of the governmental services to support older adults and their family members. This service aims to provide home-help or day care services to older adults who have trouble with independent living in order to assure security for aged citizens and also to help families with their social and economic involvements (MOHW, 2011). This service targets older adults who are not eligible for the LTC but have mild health problems or some minor levels of frailty, and whose income is less than 150% of the average for the applicable family size. It includes homemaking, meal provision, bathing, counseling and companion services, as well as home-visit nursing and day care.

Fourth is the Elderly Care Basic Service. This is a universal (not selective) program. Those aged 65 and older who live alone are eligible for this service. Income level or the existence of a legal sponsor or caregiver does not affect service eligibility. However, in order to avoid duplicate use of similar services, older adults receiving other governmental services such as the Elderly Care Comprehensive Service and the LTC do not qualify for this service. This service includes friendly check-ins (e.g., home visits once a week, phone calls more than twice a week), educational programs (e.g., promoting exercise, providing health-related information), and case management.

Although the four policies/services described above do not specifically target older adults with mental health concerns, they provide some types of help or care for those older adults. As mentioned in the previous section, there are two particular acts that aim to support people with mental health or mental health-related concerns in late life: the Dementia Management Act and the Suicide Prevention Law. Combined with the four policies/services mentioned above, these two acts are implemented at the national and local governmental levels and take into account the unique characteristics of each community.

There are few policies or services explicitly tailored to family members of older adults with mental health concerns. It is ironic that, even though the family unit has been an important feature in social welfare in Korea, a family-centered perspective in policy making is relatively new: it has attracted policymakers' attention only since the early 2000s (Chin, Lee, Lee, Son and Sung, 2012). However, policies that target older adults and their concerns still do not explicitly include family support; rather, families receive benefits indirectly or implicitly.

The Fundamental Act on Healthy Families, implemented in 2005, is the first family-centered policy focusing on the general well-being of Korean families. This Act aims to promote societal responsibility for building healthy families and communities. This act defines healthy families as ones that meet the needs of their members and promote and secure quality of life for their members. This Act creates a foundation to establish the Healthy Family Support Centers (there was a total of 152 HFSCs in 2014) which provide such services as family life education, family counseling, family-friendly community building programs, complementary child care service, emergency support for vulnerable families, and community networking (Healthy Family Support Centers, 2014). However, this Act focuses more on childcare and families with young children than it does on families with older adults who need care.

Gaps in Mental Health Policies and Services for Older Koreans

Despite recent growing public attention focused on mental health-related issues in older Koreans, social negligence and misunderstanding of these mental health concerns in later life still dominate Korean society at large. As noted earlier, people often consider older persons' mental health problems to be a part of normal ageing. There is also a tendency for older Koreans to express their psychological distresses or difficulties in the form of somatic symptoms. These tendencies contribute to under-detected and thus under-treated mental health issues among older Koreans. Public health educational programs and community-based outreach programs should be further developed to: 1) provide information on geriatric mental health conditions and formal supports available to older patients and their families; 2) identify current and/or potential patients by detecting early signs of mental disorders; and 3) develop treatment plans for these patients in a timely manner.

In response to the unprecedented growth of the older population and their increased mental health care needs, national and local governments and communities have closely worked together to help older adults and their families. Yet, the recently implemented policies and services are not sufficiently mature. For instance, the DMA provides a legal basis for preventing, identifying, and treating dementia. However, not every region in Korea benefits from this act. There are still many older patients and family members living in communities who do not have an access to social services offered by community health centers or local dementia management centers. This is often due to lack of information dissemination and insufficient staffing and/or care facilities. There is also a shortage of well-qualified or experienced professionals in this field, which often results in heavy workloads of staff members, less efficient services, and low service quality.

Another emerging issue that involves older Koreans' mental health concerns is a service area overlap. Often, disease- or problem-specific centers (e.g., dementia management centers, suicide prevention centers) are housed in local community health centers or mental health centers. Thus, multiple centers provide similar social and public health services to the same clients. Or, in these settings, the same types of care are provided to older Koreans regardless of the type of their health concerns or diagnoses. Building one-stop service centers in which older and disabled clients may obtain various needed services under the same roof has been suggested for a long time as a substitute of segregated and inefficient service provision in Korea. However, this idea has not been successfully implemented because of the hegemonic struggle between social workers and medical professionals. Recently, however, several local governments have begun to implement comprehensive services in the form of a building and/or a program as a demonstrations project to provide more integrative and preventive services to local residents.

Family members who care for older adults with mental health problems are not adequately supported by the government despite their growing needs (National Assembly Budget Office, 2014). Although formal social and public health services (e.g., day care, home-care services, short-term care services, long-term care services) have been enhanced to give better care to the increasing number of older persons with mental health problems, there are still very limited numbers of facilities and services available for family members who care for these older adults. The Fundamental Act on Healthy Families offers a basis to deliver social services to the families in need, but this act puts emphasis on families with young children and not on families with older adults who need care. A holistic service delivery approach should be carried out to include the families of vulnerable older adults.

In terms of research on geriatric mental health, there is a need to conduct nationwide epidemiological studies on mental health among older Koreans in order to estimate the prevalence of key mental disorders. In Korea, three nationwide epidemiological studies on mental illnesses have been conducted every 5 years since 2001. The most recent study, conducted in 2011, was the first that included older adults aged 65 to 74. In addition, the 2008 nationwide study on the prevalence of dementia in Korean elders was the first national epidemiological study including broader older age groups, and the second nationwide dementia study was conducted in 2012. Except for these three studies, research on geriatric mental health has been separately conducted by individual researchers and various hospitals and university research centers. Data from such research are hard to generalise to the whole older population. In order to provide valid information on mental health in older Koreans, we suggest more comprehensive research designs and initiatives that embrace researchers with multidisciplinary backgrounds and training.

Lastly, it is important to note the rapidly increasing mental health care costs of older Koreans. According to Statistics Korea (2013), the share of the National Health Insurance expenditure for the older Koreans was 33.3% although older adults account for only 12.2% of the whole population. In addition, more than 40% of LTC expenditures were spent on older adults with dementia (National Assembly Budget Office, 2014). These costs are also projected to increase with the growing number of the older population (Statistics Korea, 2013). As mentioned earlier, mental health problems in this age group are still under-detected and under-treated despite the multiple efforts in Korean society. Thus, mental health issues in older adults may need more integrative approaches, since mental health is strongly associated with, but not limited to, various physical, behavioural, and socioeconomic factors such as chronic disease, drinking behaviours, poverty, social isolation, and family conflict. More preventive and comprehensive policies or initiatives to address the needs of older adults must be considered.

Conclusion

In this chapter, we reviewed mental health issues of older Koreans and their family members. Due to the rapidly growing older population in Korea, the prevalence of several key mental health conditions like dementia and depression has been magnified as a critical social issue. In response, the Korean government has developed policies and services to help these older citizens and their families: LTC, the Elderly Care Services, the DMA, and others as described above. However, these relatively new policies and services have not yet matured. Most older adults with mental difficulties remain heavily reliant on their family members, particularly women, to provide hands-on care. Therefore, a comprehensive social support framework including the families of older Koreans with mental health concerns should be further developed. Moreover, preventive approaches to improve older adults' mental health status should be developed to facilitate the reduction of the burden of late life mental disorders. One recommendation is to encourage older Koreans to be actively engaged in social activities including working (whether paid well or not), volunteering, and enjoying leisure, as it can prevent loneliness and social isolation and improve quality of life.

References

Chang, Y. S. (2012). Trends in suicide and policy implications. *Health and Welfare Issue and Focus*, *165*, 1-8. Retrieved from https://www.kihasa.re.kr/html/jsp/publication/periodical/focus/list.jsp.

Chee, Y. K. and Levkoff, S. E. (2001). Culture and dementia: Accounts by family caregivers and health professionals for dementia-affected elders in South Korea. *Journal of Cross-Cultural Gerontology*, *16*, 111-125.

Chin, M., Lee, J., Lee, S., Son, S. and Sung, M. (2012). Family policy in South Korea: Development, current status, and challenges. *Journal of Child and Family Studies*, *21*, 53-64.

Cho, M. J., Lee, J. Y., Kim, B., Lee, H. W. and Sohn, J. H. (2011). Prevalence of the major mental disorders among the Korean elderly. *Journal of Korean Medical Science*, *26*, 1-10.

Cho, M. J. and Sohn, J. (2013). Geriatric psychiatric research in Korea. In S. Choi, J. Bae, K. Min, Y. Roh and Y. Won (Eds.), *Ageing in Korea* (pp. 212-247). Seoul, Republic of Korea: Federation of Korean Gerontological Societies.

Choi, S. J. (2009). Ageing society issues in Korea. *Asian Social Work and Policy Review, 3*, 63-83.

Goldsmith, R. L. (2012). Health care system structure and delivery in the Republic of Korea: Considerations for health care reform implementation in the United States. 30-41. Retrieved from http://www.sppa.udel.edu/sites/sppa.udel.edu/files/pdf/NVPA_Linstead_Goldsmith_2012.pdf.

Healthy Family Support Center (2014). *Current National Healthy Family Support Centers*. Retrieved Sep 10, 2014, from http://www. familynet.or.kr/.

Jeon, H. J. (2011). Depression and suicide. *Journal of Korean Medical Association*, *54*(4), 370-375.

Jones, R. S. (2010). Health care reform in Korea. Economic Department Working Papers No. 797. Organization for Economic Co-operation and Development. Retrieved from www.oecd.org/workingpapers.

Jung, K. (2013). Review of the current policies and policy agenda regarding elder abuse. *Health and Welfare Forum*, *200*, 51-61. Retrieved from https://www.kihasa.re.kr/html/jsp/publication/periodical/forum/view.jsp?bid=19&aid=262&ano=297.

Jung, K., Oh, Y., Lee, Y., Son, C., Park, B. and Lee, S. (2012). National survey of senior citizen 2011. Korean Institute for Health and Social Affairs and Ministry of Health and Welfare. Retrieved from http://stat.mw.go.kr/front/include/download.jsp?bbsSeq=7&nttSeq=20275&atchSeq=3318.

Kessler, R. C., Chiu, W. T., Demler, O., Merikangas, K. R. and Walters, E. E. (2005). Prevalence, severity, and comorbidity of 12-month DSM-IV disorders in the national comorbidity survey replication. *Archives of General Psychiatry*, *62*, 617-627.

Kim, B., Lee, D., Bae, J. N., Chang, S. M., Kim, S., Kim, K. W., Rim, H., Park, J. E. and Cho, M. J., (2014). Impact of illiteracy on depression symptomatology in community-dwelling older adults. *International Psychogeriatrics*, *26*(10), 1669-1678.

Kim, E. H. and Cook, P. J. (2011). The continuing importance of children in relieving elder poverty: evidence from Korea. *Ageing and Society*, *31*, 953-976.

Kim, K. N., Kim, C. H., Kim, K. I., Yoo, H. J., Park, S. Y. and Park, Y. H. (2012). Development and validation of the Korean nursing delirium scale. *Journal of Korean Academy of Nursing*, *42*(3), 414-423.

Kim, K. W., Park, J. H., Kim, M., Kim, M. D., Kim, B. and Kim, S. (2011). A nationwide survey on the prevalence of dementia and mild cognitive impairment in South Korea. *Journal of Alzheimer's Disease*, *23*, 281-291.

Kim, S. H. and Han, S. (2012). Prevalence of dementia among the South Korean population. *Journal of Korean Diabetes*, *13*, 124-128.

Kim, Y. J., Han, J. W., So, Y. S., Seo, J. Y., Kim, K. Y. and Kim, K. W. (2014). Prevalence and trends of dementia in Korea: A systematic review and meta-analysis. *Journal of Korean Medical Science*, *29*, 903-912.

Kinsella, K. and He, W. (2009). An aging world: 2008 *International Population Reports*. Washington, DC: National Institute on Aging and U.S. Census Bureau.

Knight, B. G., Robinson, G. S., Flynn Longmire, C., Chun, M., Nakao, K. and Kim, J. H. (2002). Cross cultural issues in caregiving for dementia: Do familism values reduce burden and distress? *Ageing International*, *27*, 70-93.

Ko, K. D., Cho, Y. T., Cho, S. I., Sung, J. H., Cho, B. L., Son, K. Y. and Choi, H. C. (2012). Association of health risk behaviors with mental health among elderly Koreans. *Journal of Korean Geriatric Society*, *16*(2), 66-73.

Korea Institute for Health and Social Affairs (KIHASA). (2006). The elderly care insurance pilot study evaluation report. Ministry of Health and Welfare. Korea Institute for Health and Social Affairs. Retrieved from http://repository.kihasa.re.kr:8080/handle/201002/1651.

Korea Institute for Health and Social Affairs (KIHASA). (2010). *The 2009 National Elder Abuse Incidence Study*. Ministry of Health and Welfare. Korea Institute for Health and Social Affairs.

Korea Suicide Prevention Center (2014). Current statistics of suicide. Retrieved from http://www.spckorea.or.kr/.

Korean Statistical Information Service (KOSIS). (2014). Population by census. Retrieved June 2, 2014 from http://kosis.kr/.

Lee, M., Yoon, E. and Kropf, N. (2007). Factors affecting burden of South Koreans providing care to disabled older family members. *International Journal of Aging and Human Development*, *64*(3), 245-262.

Lee, M. S., Choi, Y. K., Jung, I. K. and Kwak, D. I. (2000). Epidemiological study of geriatric depression in a Korea urban area. *Journal of Korean Geriatric Psychiatry*, *4*(2), 154-163.

McLean, C. P., Asnaani, A., Litz, B. T. and Hofmann, S. G. (2011). Gender differences in anxiety disorders: Prevalence, course of illness, comorbidity and burden of illness. *Journal of Psychiatric Research*, *45*(8), 1027-1035.

Ministry of Health and Welfare (2011).Guide to the elderly care services, *2011*. Daejeon: Ministry of Health and Welfare. Retrieved from http://www.socialservice.or.kr/upload/etc/2014_1000.pdf.

Ministry of Health and Welfare (2014). Guide to mental health services, 2014. Daejeon: Ministry of Health and Welfare. Retrieved from http://www.mw.go.kr/.

National Assembly Budget Office (2014). Evaluation and policy recommendation on the dementia management service. Retrieved from http://www.nabo.go.kr/index.jsp.

OECD (2013). *Health at a glance 2013: OECD indicators*. Paris: OECD Publishing. Retrieved from http://dx.doi.org/10.1787/health_glance-2013-71-en.

Oh, D. H., Park, J. H., Lee, H. Y., Kim, S. A., Choi, B. Y. and Nam, J. H. (2014). Association between living arrangements and depressive symptoms among older women and men in South Korea. *Social Psychiatry and Psychiatric Epidemiology*, *50*(1), 133-141.

Oh, Y. (2013). Elderly health and policy implications. Health and Welfare Issue and Focus, 220, 1-8. Seoul: Korean Institute for Health and Social Affairs. Retrieved from https://www.kihasa.re.kr/html/jsp/share/download_forum.jsp?bid=21&aid=292&ano=386.

Park, J. H., Lee, J. J., Lee, S. B., Huh, Y., Choi, E. A. and Youn, J. C. (2010). Prevalence of major depressive disorder and minor depressive disorder in an elderly Korean population: Results from the Korean Longitudinal Study on Health and Aging (KLoSHA). *Journal of Affective Disorders*, *125*(1-3), 234-240.

Seoul National University Hospital (2009). *The Nationwide Study on the Prevalence of Dementia in Korean Elders: Final Report.* Seoul: Seoul National University Hospital.

Seoul National University Hospital (2011). *The Epidemiological Survey of Mental Disorders in Korea.* Seoul: Seoul National University Hospital.

Shin, S. and Lukens, E. P. (2002). Effects of psychoeducation for Korean Americans with chronic mental illness. *Psychiatric Services*, *53*(9), 1125-1131. Retrieved from http://ps.psychiatryonline.org/article.aspx? articleid=180401.

Statistical Research Institute (2007). Trends in elderly suicide and cause analysis. Daejeon: Statistical Research Institute. Retrieved from http://kostat.go.kr/edu/sri_kor_new/1/1/index.action?bmode=download&p_idx=61.

Statistics Korea (2011). Population projections for Korea: 2010-2060 (Based on the 2010 Census). Daejeon: Statistics Korea. Retrieved from http://kosis.kr/ups/ups_01List01.jsp?pubcode=PJ#.

Statistics Korea (2013). The 2013 elderly statistics. Retrieved from http://kostat.go.kr/.

Sung, K. (2001). Family support for the elderly in Korea. *Journal of Aging and Social Policy*, *12*(4), 65-79.

In: Ageing and Mental Health: Global Perspectives
Editors: Wendy Wen Li, Sherry M. Cummings et al.
ISBN: 978-1-63484-777-3

Chapter 8

SOCIAL CARE FOR OLDER ADULTS WITH MENTAL DISORDER IN JAPAN

Hiroko Kase*
Waseda University, Tokyo, Japan

ABSTRACT

In 2007, when the percentage of the population aged 65 or older had reached 21.5%, Japan was designated a 'super-aged' society. The Long-Term Care Insurance (LTCI), the nationally mandated long-term care insurance programme for older adults, had already been implemented by the government in 2000. This system changed the public's understanding of social care, which had previously been regarded as a service for the poor, to that of a social service available for all Japanese citizens. The Act on Service and Support for Persons with Disabilities (ASSPD), including mental disorders, approved in 2006, integrated social services and public medical services that had previously been provided, based on different laws for different disabilities, following the same ideas and systems of the LTCI programme.

The present chapter discusses the current services and policies and how they relate to older Japanese individuals with mental illness. It emphasises the importance of re-evaluating the kinds of care that should be provided and under what circumstances. Additionally, future risks to the stability of the social security system as a result of the ageing society are also considered. The sustainability of long-term care and home care, mainly provided by family care givers, is perhaps the issue most in need of being addressed by both regional and national governments at the present time.

Keywords: family care giving, long-term care, mental health, older adults, community-based care

* Corresponding author: Hiroko Kase, email: hkase@waseda.jp.

Introduction

After the Second World War, Japan embarked on a path to establish itself as a welfare state, with its Constitution making provision for maintaining minimum standards of wholesome and cultured living for its citizens. (Ministry of Justice, 2015a). Japan had rapidly established the policies and systems of social security and welfare, with an average annual GDP growth of 10% between 1955 and 1973 (Cabinet Office, 2015a). This same period of rapid industrialisation pre-empted the emergence of the 'nuclear family', as well as a shift from rural areas to urban areas by the younger population, and the subsequent collapse of traditional family care for older adults. In 1963, the Act on Social Welfare for the Elderly was implemented in order to provide services for all older adults, as well as institutional care in public nursing homes (*tokubetu yogo roujin* homes) (Ministry of Justice, 2015b). However the social care services made available by this act applied only to those older adults on low incomes who were living alone. Kasza (2006) made a salient point by saying that the Japanese formula for economic success was to minimize spending on anything that diverted resources from industrial investment, including spending on public welfare.

The medical conditions and welfare of older adults during the 1970s made the need for immediate reforms apparent. A national survey conducted in 1968 by the Japan National Council of Social Welfare estimated that 17% of the aged population was bedridden, a percentage which alarmed bureaucrats at the Ministry of Health and Welfare (MHW) (Campbell, 1993). Approximately 42% of the bedridden elderly, estimated at 250,000, had previously been cared for at hospitals, while 230,000 older people had been cared for by family at their own homes. (Showa 63 Nendo Kosei Kagaku Tokubetu Kenkyu Jigyo, 2003). Due to the shortage of nursing facilities, as well as the stigma associated with being cared for at *tokubetu yogo roujin* homes (public nursing homes), the urgent need to address the growing demand for elderly care in hospitals became apparent. Although out-of-pocket expenses for patients had reduced from 50% to 30% of total medical costs under the revision of the National Health Insurance Act (NHI) (National Institute of Population and Social Security Research, 2014), many older citizens could no longer afford to use such medical services (Tsumura, 1973). In response, almost all major prefectural governments, including the Tokyo metropolitan government, established a free medical care system for older adults, with the national government following suit. In 1972, the Act on Social Welfare for the Elderly was amended, requiring the national government to exempt out-of-pocket expenses for older adults and ensure complete health insurance coverage for all aged 70 and older, and those aged 65-69 who were bedridden (Ministry of Health, Labor and Welfare, 2007).

This free medical care system resulted in an increased demand for medical care and a sudden increase in hospitalisation of older adults, not only those who were bedridden, but also those who were not in need of medical treatment but needed care of various kinds for an indefinite period of time (Estevez-Abe, 2007).

As can be seen in Figure 1, from 1977 onward, the place where Japanese citizens died shifted markedly from homes to hospitals.

Neither the significant cost factor nor the consequences on traditional family care structure, had been anticipated at the national level. For both economic and social reasons, possibly stemming from a certain neo-capitalist trend triggered by the oil crisis, as well as concerns about shifts in family structure, a directive of welfare retrenchment was given by the national government, emphasising community-based care over institutional care. Early in the 1980s, The National Council for Social Welfare recommended that, as a principle of policy, the national government should establish home-based services, which were previously considered supplementary to institutional care. The Council also recommended "changes to the social welfare system so as to provide services for all older adults, regardless of income" (Chuo Shakai Fukushi Shingikai, 1981, p. 3, Author's own translation). There was, however, no noticeable increase in either the number of users or the number of hours of home help service provided, though home helpers increased by 3,298 in 1982 (Suga, 1996).

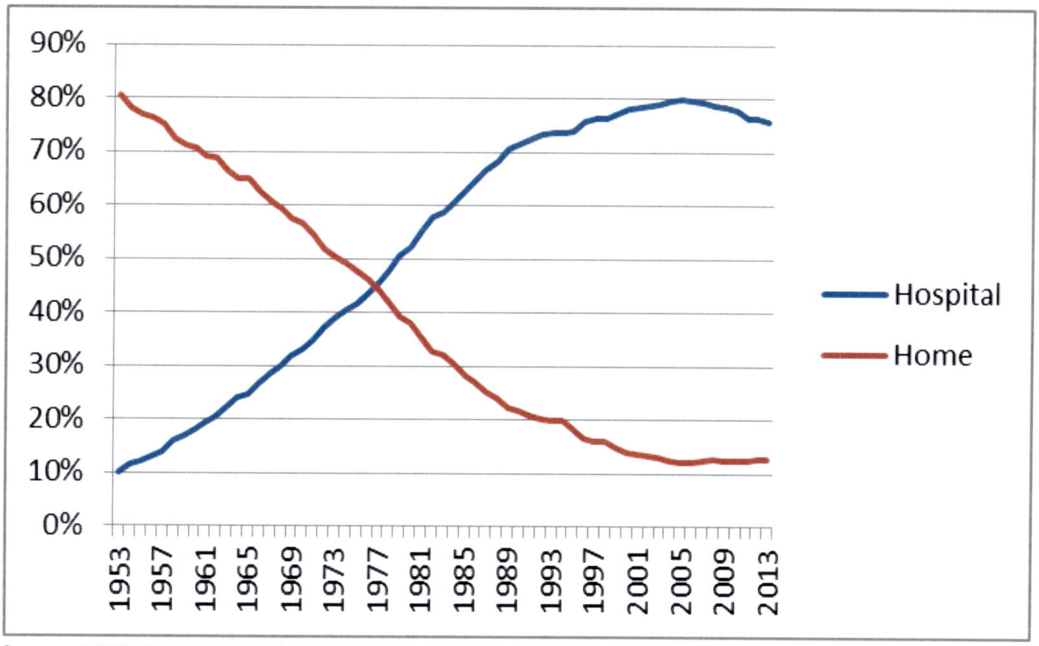

Source: MHLW, Demographic survey 2014.

Figure 1 Location of deaths in Japan 1953-2013.

The impetus which led to a major increase in community-based services came from outside of the sphere of welfare policy reform, when, in 1988, the Consumption Tax Act was discussed in parliament (Administration Bureau, 2015a). Using part of the revenue made available by the consumption tax, 'The Strategy for Elderly Persons' Health and Welfare Promotion over the Next Ten Years' (The Gold Plan) was implemented, ushering in an increase in general services provided to older adults in need of nursing. It was expected that the 'Gold Plan' would provide for an expenditure of ￥6 trillion (US$60 billion) over the following ten years, and would bolster the goals and utilisation of the three main community-based services: home help services, short stay services, and adult day care services (MHW, 1989).

Home help services provides funding for home visits by personal care and housekeeping service professionals; short stay services provides for one week or two weeks respite care in a public nursing home; and adult day care services provides for group activities at a facility in the community in order to promote independence in carrying out activities of daily living and better mental health. In addition, the visiting-nurse system, which allowed registered nurses to establish 'visiting-nurse (*homon kango*) stations' as private businesses commenced in 1991. Such progress in providing welfare for older people, together with the community-based care surge, presented a previously neglected area of opportunity for business, namely, the private sector. Privatisation has been accelerated under the Long-term Care Insurance since 2000.

Mental Health Problems in Older People

When the proportion of the population aged 65 and older reached 21.5% in 2007 (Cabinet Office, 2008), Japan became regarded as a 'super-aged' society. According to the Statistics Bureau in the Ministry of Internal Affairs and Communications, in October of 2014, the number of people aged 65 and older reached a record high of 33 million, comprising 26% of the total population (Statistics Bureau, 2015a). Regarding the future, it is estimated that the dependency ratio of elderly people to working-age people will continue to rise, reaching 40.5% in 2055, when there will be one elderly person for every 1.3 working-aged people. (Table 1).

Mental health is a significant issue among Japanese older adults and their families. The existence of senile dementia was already well known by the public through literature and films, for example, the novel named *Koukotu no hito,* meaning a person in rapture, described a portrayal of man who suffered from dementia and his struggling family, became a best seller book in 1972 (MacDonald, 2008).

Table 1. Japan's Population Profile, 1950~2055

		1950	1975	2009	2030	2055
Population (1000)	All ages	84,115	111,940	127,510	115,224	89,930
	0-14 years old	29,786	27,221	17,011	11,150	7,516
	15-64 years old	50,168	75,807	81,493	67,404	45,951
	65 and over	4,155	8,865	29,005	36,670	36,463
Age structure	0-14 years old	35.40%	24.30%	13.30%	9.70%	8.40%
	15-64 years old	59.60%	67.70%	63.90%	58.50%	51.10%
	65 and over	4.90%	7.90%	22.80%	31.80%	40.50%
Fertility	Total fertility rate	3.65	1.91	1.37		-
Life expectancy	Male	*59.57	71.73	79.59	-	-
	Female	*62.97	76.89	86.44	-	-

Note: Data with * are those of averages from 1950 to 1952 (Figures may not add up to the totals because of rounding).

Source: NIPSSR, *Social Security in Japan 2011* (p. 3).

The estimated numbers of mental disorder patients in Japan are shown in Figure 2. Patients with mental health disorders associated with Alzheimer's disease and cerebrovascular dementia are predominantly elderly, and predominantly female.

The proportion of patients with mental disorders in the over 65 population is shown in Figure 3. The number of dementia patients, combining those with vascular dementia and Alzheimer's patients, is only 2% of the aged population. However this figure represents only the number of patients who have been diagnosed. The Ministry of Health, Law and Welfare (MHLW) estimates that the more accurate percentage would be between 8 to 10% (MHLW,

2015a). These facts suggest that less than 20% of people suffering from dementia have been diagnosed as such.

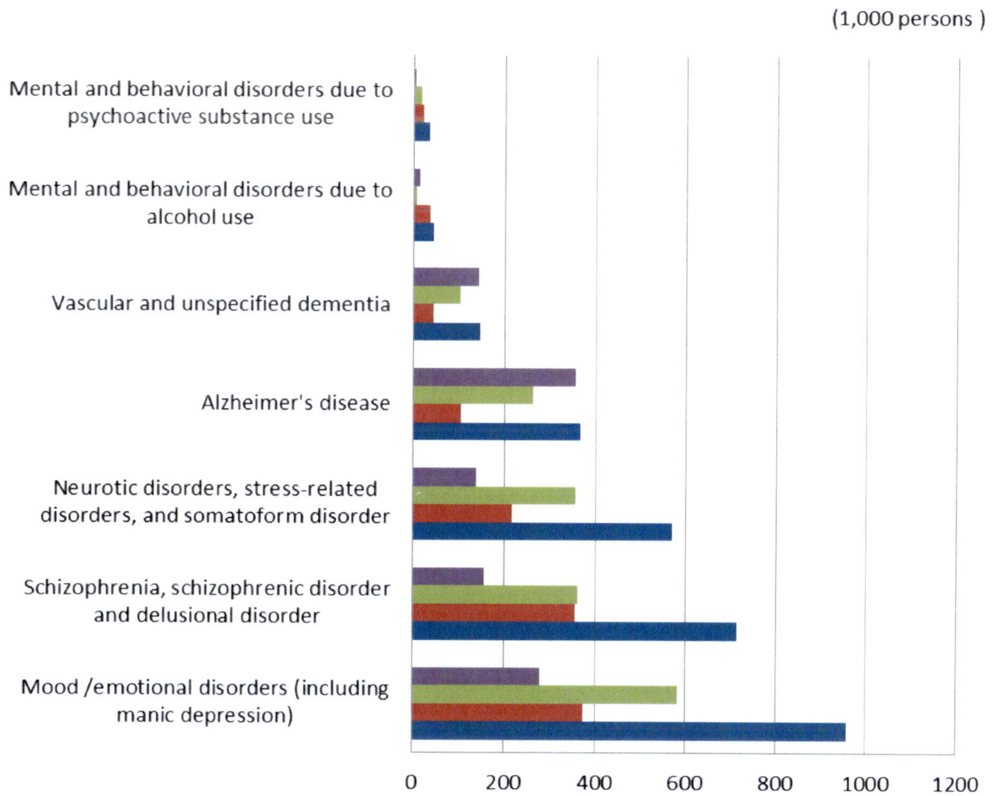

	Mood /emotional disorders (including manic depression)	Schizophrenia, schizophrenic disorder and delusional disorder	Neurotic disorders, stress-related disorders, and somatoform disorder	Alzheimer's disease	Vascular and unspecified dementia	Mental and behavioral disorders due to alcohol use	Mental and behavioral disorders due to psychoactive substance use
65 and over	278	155	138	356	142	13	3
female	584	360	356	262	103	7	15
male	374	354	215	104	43	36	20
total	958	713	571	366	146	43	35

Source: MHLW, Patient Survey 2011.

Figure 2. Prevalence of mental disorders.

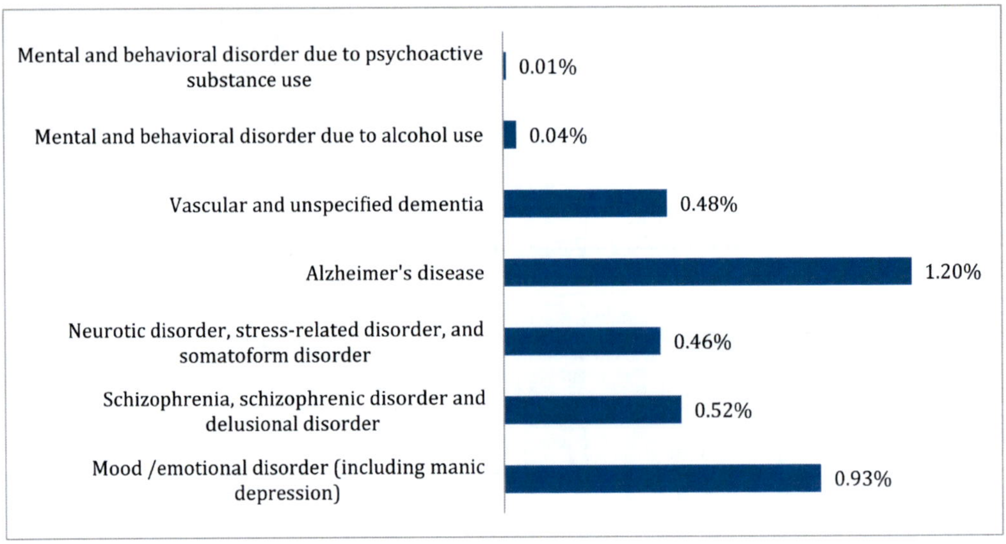

Source: MHLW, Patient Survey (kanja chousa) 2011.

Figure 3. Mental disorder patients as a percentage of aged population in 2011.

In Japan, it has traditionally been the role of women to look after family members, and as recent as 2013, it was established that 70% of main family caregivers who care for older adults are women (MHLW, 2013a). However, lower mortality rates, combined with rapid urbanisation, and changing living arrangements, may also contribute to this percentage. For example, 3 million elderly people, representing 6% of all households, were living alone in 2000. It is estimated, however, that by 2020, 6.3 million people, representing 12.5% of all households, will be older adults living alone (Cabinet Office, 2012).

LONG-TERM CARE INSURANCE (LTCI)

The national government implemented the Long-Term Care Insurance (*kaigo hoken*) as the nationally mandated long-term care insurance programme for older adults in 2000 (Ministry of Justice, 2015c). This system resulted in a change in the public's understanding of social care, which had previously been regarded as a service for the poor. The LTCI provides for community care such as home helpers, visiting nurses and day care services, as well as institutionalised care such as senior health care homes and nursing homes. The LTCI only covers costs related to the care of older adults, with no provision made for younger persons with disabilities. Unlike many other developed countries, provisions for community-based care in Japan is double-tiered, namely, it is provided by the LTCI Act, and also by the Services and Support for Persons with Disabilities Act, which was enacted to ensure consistency with the LTCI (Ministry of Justice, 2015d). Those entitled to coverage by the LTCI are adults aged 65 and older (Category I), in addition to subscribers to health insurance who are 40 to 64 years of age (Category II). Those eligible to receive long-term care include all persons in Category I who are certified as needing support or nursing care based on examination by the Certification Committee for Long-Term Care Need (MHLW, 2015b). For Category II persons, care is limited to individuals requiring nursing care or support due to age-related diseases such as dementia and cerebrovascular disorders. In addition to co-payment by users, 50% of the cost of care services is financed by premiums paid for by everyone over age 40; 20% from Category I persons and 30% from Category II persons, with the remaining 50% financed by public expenditures. The estimated average cost for an older adult, from 2000 to 2002, was approximately ¥2,900 (approximately US$29) per month. Between 2009 and 2011, the average amount had increased to ¥4,160 (US$42) per month. The amount of co-payment for care services is fixed for both Category I persons and Category II persons at 10% of the total cost of services, with users required to bear the cost of meals and expenses in the facilities, such as accommodation utilities (National Institute of Population and Social Security Research, 2011).

As of 2015, service-users are classified into seven levels depending on the nature of the care needs, as determined by municipal assessment, which is a prerequisite for having such services provided. Upon receipt of an application, a municipal assessor visits the applicant's home for an interview to evaluate his or her physical and mental state, and aspects of daily life (MHLW, 2015c). In practice, the interview is carried out using a unified form, nationwide, with the primary evaluation being reached using a computer algorithm for the 74 questions on the form. The needs assessment is determined on the basis of a national standard, not a local decision, such as that made in the UK or Sweden. Even the review of the decision is made by an independent Certification Committee for Long-Term Care Need, which is appointed by the mayor in the municipality, but which is unrelated to local government. Once the category of needed care assistance has been determined, each service-user chooses a care manager who draws up an individualised care plan and helps coordinate the necessary services for the service-user. Service-users can choose from among services which remain within the limits of the amount allowable for their care need level and care plan. In order to be certified as a care manager, a person must have had five-year-experience in community based care as a professional, such as a nurse, a certified care worker, a certified social worker or other such care-work professionals. They are then required to pass a national examination and complete a nationally authorised programme of training by the LTCI Act Article 69. (Ministry of Justice, 2015c). Most care managers are employees of the Home Care Support Office which is under private sector management. The number of cases assigned to each care manager is limited to no more than 43 (including 8 preventive care level cases) as stipulated under the law.

Strategies for the Long-Term Care Insurance Reform

In the year 2000, when the LTCI was first implemented, the total cost of such care was ¥3.6 trillion (US$36 billion). However the increasing number of institutionalised users covered by the LTCI resulted in a significant increase in the cost of long term care, and by 2007, it had increased to ¥7.1 trillion (US$71 billion). To address this burgeoning expenditure, the subsequent 2005 reform of the LTCI Act placed greater emphasis on community-based services to be managed and supervised at the local level by municipalities, anticipating that such a delivery system would reduce costs (MHLW, 2005a). In contrast to the plan for the earlier 'Japanese-Style Welfare Society' model, the MHLW introduced the new idea of a mutual help system which would supplement long-term care services in the community. The main purpose of this strategy is to organise social support networks to provide support for older adults living in the community. To promote such social support networks, drawing on the support from volunteers, neighbours and social resources in the community, the national government requires each municipality to establish Community General Support Centers (CGSC) for older people, with each serving from between 3,000 to 6,000 seniors. According to national guidelines, each CGSC is expected to contribute to the implementation of preventive care management (maintaining activities of daily living) to provide comprehensive consulting and support, such as providing advocacy for vulnerable persons and to help care managers deliver 'Comprehensive and Continuing (*houkatsuteki/keizokuteki)* Care Management'. Each CGSC is required to have a public health nurse, a certified social worker, and a care management supervisor. Under the direction of the MHLW, municipalities and local CGSCs are required to organize so- called 'informal networks' in the communities to promote mutual help (*kyojo*). The MHLW has promoted a campaign to establish a community network movement to assist people with dementia (*ninchisho mimamor*i network) and staff of the CGSCs are mobilised to recruit volunteers to help the frail elderly in the community. The idea is that relatively younger elders, notably the 'baby boomers', would become a supportive resource for the 'super-aged' society.

Historically in Japan, local residents align their lifestyle to suit gaps in public welfare policy. In the mid-1900s, the Japanese government adopted a volunteer system, modelled on a parish in Germany, to look after people experiencing poverty (Chibaken Minji Kyo, 2015). This initiative marked the start of the home-visit volunteer (*homen iin*) system, which was subsequently incorporated into the commissioned welfare volunteer (*minsei iin*) system, under the Commissioned Welfare Volunteers Law of 1948 (Zenkoku Minsei Iin Jidou Iin Rengoukai, 2015). The CGSCs relied considerably on the volunteer services of the *minsei iin*. However it was unable to recruit a sufficient number of new volunteers from among the relatively younger people in older adult age group, even though most of the *minsei iin* were middle aged or elderly. The only movement to have succeeded is the Supporter System for People with Dementia, which offers a one-hour lecture about dementia. It became popular among people who had a specific interest in dementia and in obtaining certification as a supporter for those with dementia (*ninchishou* supporters). The number of those who joined this movement, and who attended lectures, was about 6,018,000, as of 2015 (Zenkoku Caravan Meito Renraku Kyougikai, 2015). The MHLW has campaigned to promote 'Orange Café' for people with dementia run by volunteers and the supporters and their family care givers since 2013. The emergence of volunteer groups in the community to help people with dementia, however, has yet to be seen in most cases, suggesting that simply attending a lecture, by itself, does not result in attracting people to commit to volunteer care provision in local communities.

INCREASING DISPARITY AMONG PRIVATE FACILITIES

The MHLW only approves applications for the construction of new public nursing homes which have care units for a small number of residents living in single rooms, even in a large facility under the LTCI. This model of small group care, called 'unit care', has been selected because it is thought that it would create a more home-like atmosphere. However, the average cost of a single room with meals is approximately ￥60,000 (US$600) per month, to be paid by the resident. Those who could not afford the room and board fee would have to wait for a vacancy in older facilities which offers four beds sharing units. This causes municipality officials in the Tokyo area to send public users seeking assistance to unapproved care facilities in rural cities which sometimes do not meet minimum safety requirements. One such facility had confined elderly patients with dementia to their rooms. As a result, when a fire broke out in March, 2009, 10 residents died. Despite such safety hazards, only 40% of elderly public assistance users who require institutional care can be accommodated in public nursing homes in Tokyo, with the remaining 60%, or 1,785 of elderly public assistance users, needing to be referred to rural areas. Compared with the number of such referrals in January 2009, the number had doubled for November of same year. (Itou, 2013).

Due to the shortage of public nursing homes and the increasing need for dementia care, the MHLW in 2005 established group homes for people with dementia. Residents in these facilities would need to provide an additional payment of approximately ￥100,000 (US$1,000) per month. Additionally, in 2005, another special private facility (*tokutei shisetsu*) was introduced. It also requires users to pay extra, bringing the cost up to more than ￥250,000 (US$2,500) per month. The additional cost provides for a broad range of services as such facilities are designated as being community-based services under the LTCI which offer a variety of accommodation choices with regard to both space and quality. Many of these private facilities function like a nursing facility. However the LTCI covers only the costs required for ordinary care. The cost of construction and of additional personnel, which is usually covered by public funds in public nursing facilities, is covered by service-users in these new private facilities. Similarly since 2011, the Ministry of Land, Infrastructure, Transport and Tourism, has promoted the construction of apartments for seniors with supportive services, such as information and referral services (Sabisu Tuki Koureisya Muki Jyutaku, 2015).

MENTAL HEALTH CARE REFORM

The development of community mental health care began in 2002, stemming from a MHLW report called 'The Future Direction of Mental Health and Welfare Policy.' This 'Reform Vision' report fundamentally addressed the shift from hospital-based medical treatment to community-centred health care and welfare. The overall aim of the report was to realise the transition from institution-based medical treatment to community-based care (Chuo Shakai Hoshou Singikai Shougaisya Bukai Seishin Syougai Bunkai, 2002). To achieve the objectives of the Reform Vision, definitive goals for the next 10 years were set for public education and for the mental health care system. The reform process, aimed at reducing the number of hospital beds by 70,000 within 10 years, had a considerable impact on the subsequent approach to community mental health care. In 2006, the Act on Services and Supports for Persons with Disabilities, which was amended in 2012, integrated both social services and public medical services that had previously been provided based on different laws for different disabilities (Administration Bureau, 2015b). It followed the same ideas and systems of the LTCI, including the classification of disabilities, Community Life Support Centre, and the requirement of a 10% co-payment. Many professionals and practitioners working in community and hospital sectors struggled to cope with this major change, which was a significant step towards the realisation of a community-based mental health care system. In 1965, the number of people with mental health needs who lived in hospitals was 177,170. This increased to 348,859 in 1990, and then decreased to 311,007 in 2010 after the reforms had been implemented (MHLW, 2015d). Notwithstanding the emphasis placed on community care, there was no major decrease in the number of hospitalised patients in need of mental health care. In 2011, the average length of hospitalisation in mental hospitals was 389.8 days, which was 101.7 days shorter than in 1996, but improvement has not been significant (Figure 4).

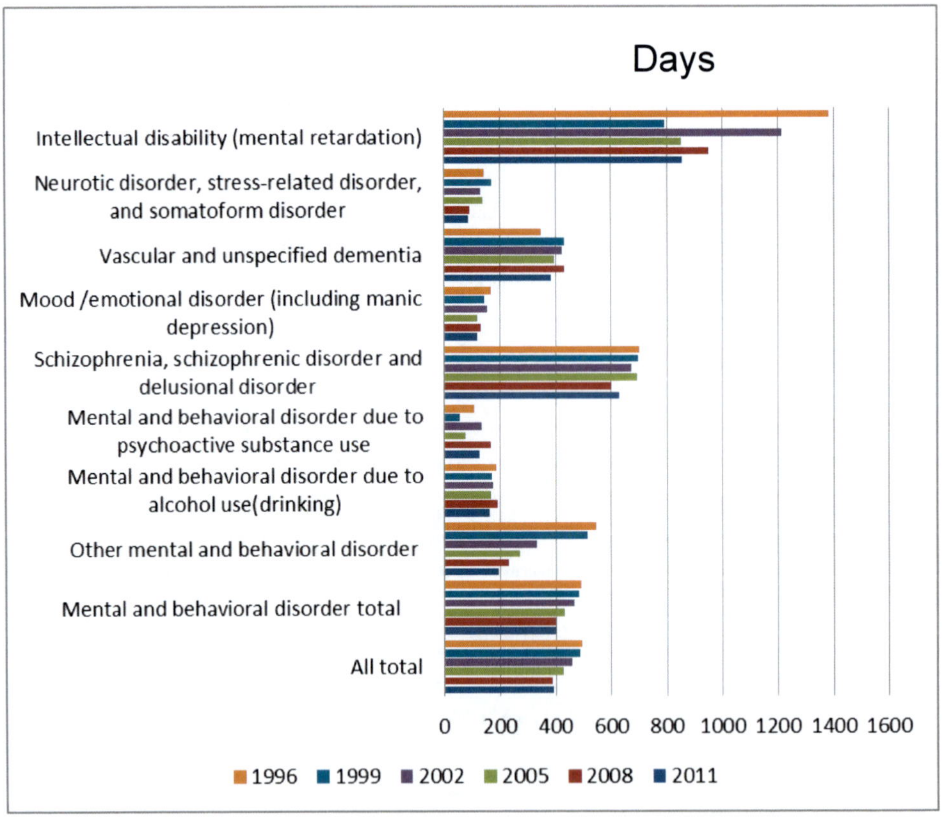

Source: MHLW, Patient Survey (kanjya chousa) 2011, 2008, 2005b, 2002, 1999, 1996.

Figure 4. Average length of hospitalization in mental hospitals.

Social Care Services for Older Adults with Mental Disorders

In this section, a case study is presented so as to present the real issues facing older adults with mental and physical health problems in Japan.

Case Study

Mrs. H was born at a location about 100km north of Tokyo, and raised as the second of four children by merchant parents. In a city close to central Tokyo, Mrs. H and her husband established a small shop selling stationary and snacks, mainly for high school students. She dealt with the management and accounting of their business. Her hobbies included singing karaoke and performing Japanese traditional dance.

In 1995, Mrs. H suffered a cerebral infarction which paralysed the left side of her body in 1995. With her dedication to rehabilitation, she recovered sufficiently as to be able to enjoy vacations several times a year. She could walk with a cane and was able to use public transportation, but needed training on how to maintain her daily living activities due to her declining physical strength. She started rehabilitation once a week at an adult day care centre under the LTCI in April 2005. The adult day care centre functions like an adult day service centre, but has to have the services of a physical therapist or an occupational therapist. Mrs. H completed this training programme and was stable in her physical and mental condition. Thus the case was closed at the end of September 2010. In April 2011, however, she was hospitalised for 14 days having been diagnosed with a duodenal ulcer. The extended period of recovery in bed caused difficulty in walking.

At 82 years old, and categorised at care need level 5 (bedridden) by the LTCI, she is unable to walk and is bedridden at home, except for attendance at an adult day care centre once a week with the help of a wheelchair. She uses adult diapers at all times and requires full assistance with eating, bathing, and changing clothes, but is able to hold a normal conversation. Mrs. H lives with her 84 year-old husband and their 55 year-old son. Her husband has suffered from lower back pain since he was young, and was diagnosed with spinal column stenosis in his 60s. He is categorised at care need level 2 by the LTCI due to lumbar spinal canal stenosis. Mrs. H told the care manager that her son was also suffering from dysautonomia and had changed his job many times. Her son goes to work early in the morning every day and is not well informed about his parents' conditions.

Mrs. H chose her former care manager, a certified social worker, to create a care plan when she became a service-user of the LTCI again, in May 2011. The care manager developed a care plan for Mrs. H with the goal of reducing the burden of care on her husband, and also ensuring she could receive ongoing care in their own home. The weekly care plan included adult day service from 9 a.m.to 4 p.m. once a week, home help service three times a day(except week-end), from 9:00-9:30, 12:30-13:00, 17:30-18:00 for changing her diapers and assisting her with meals, and a visit by a nurse once a week for a medical check, medication management, and emptying her bowels by enema. Mrs. H needed an electric bed and a mat to prevent bed sores, and a wheelchair for going out. Also she was not able to use a normal bathtub. Therefore, the care manager proposed using a visiting bathing service in which a provider brings a special flat bathtub for bedridden people into her home once a week. The cost was ¥12,000 (US$120) per day for adult day service, ¥2,900 (US$29) per time for home help, ¥8,000 per visit by a nurse, ¥12,500 (US$125) per time for assisted bathing, with a rental fee of ¥13,000 per month for a bed with matt and a wheelchair. The total cost was estimated to be ¥325,700 per month (US$3,257), with an expected co-payment of ¥ 32,740 per month. Mr. and Mrs. H's total household income was approximately ¥80,000 per month by pension, since they had only contributed minimum pension premiums, being small independent business owners.

The care manager recognised that Mrs. H had risks of dehydration as she had superficial anaesthesia due to her brain condition. As such, included into her care was the need for the home helpers to keep her hydrated during their visits through different ways including making jelly with sweet juice. However, Mrs. H could only imbibe 250ml to 500ml of water a day. The home helpers also reported to the care manger that Mrs. H was always complaining about feeling cold, and always requiring additional blankets. She also sometimes refused to eat. As a result of dehydration and poor nutrition, Mrs. H was hospitalised one year later in 2013 for 15 days due to high fever and cognitive confusion. A hospital stay of this length for dehydration is unusual under the NHI, but unfortunately her husband was also staying at the hospital at the same time due to his propensity to fall. Since her son was unable to take care of her, she decided to use a private room and paid an additional fee of ¥15,000 (US$150) per day, making it possible for her to stay at the hospital. Subsequently, a medical (health) social worker at the hospital recommended having the support of a home doctor and introduced a visiting physician after Mrs. H. was discharged. The care manager then added an additional visit by a doctor per month to the care plan. The cost of this came up to ¥12,000 (US$120) per month which was covered by the NHI, with an estimated co-payment of ¥1,200 (US$12) per month.

By August 2013, Mrs. H had become obsessed with the idea that her neighbours were making disparaging remarks about her. The visiting physician called the care manager and advised him to arrange for a psychiatrist to assess the status of her mental health. The care manager visited Mrs. H and her husband to discuss their options and recommended the services of the Outpatient Psychiatric Care Services under the Services and Supports for Persons with Disabilities Act (SSPDA). This would allow Mrs. H to have more frequent visits by a psychiatrist and lower out-of-pocket payments than under the LTCI. However, Mr. and Mrs. H said they disliked having to pay more for care services and did not want more people coming into their house. From December 2012 to September 2014, the care manager arranged interdisciplinary meetings between Mrs. H and her family and social and health care professionals, including a public health nurse from the city office and a social worker from CGSC.

In October 2014, the application written by the care manager on behalf of Mrs. H was accepted by the municipality, enabling Mrs. H to use services provided for by SSPDA. A psychiatrist diagnosed her as having depression and prescribed medication. The treatment was effective and helped to reduce her delusions and increased her appetite.

In sum, Mrs. H now uses care services covered by the LTCI, Home Visiting Medical Care covered by the NHI, and Outpatient Psychiatric Care Service which provides two visits per month by a psychiatrist, covered by SSPDA. The total monthly cost of all these services is estimated to be ¥409,400 (US$4,094), with a co-payment of ¥40,940 (US$409) which is equal to a half of total monthly income of Mr. and Mrs. H.

GAPS AND CHALLENGES

While the LTCI has made long-term care services available to a larger number of people and broadened the range of services provided, it remains to be seen whether the privatisation of the LTCI is efficient and effective. There is a need to provide the LTCI services that improve the quality of life of its service-users and give providers flexibility in working with family care givers. In spite of considerable efforts made to reduce the burden of family care givers, a national survey shows that 35.9% of them spent "almost a whole day" taking care of older adults classified as at level 3, 53.9% for level 4, and 56.1% for level 5. It also indicated that 61.6% of main care givers are family members living with older adults in need, while 9.6% are those living separately. Only 14.8% are service providers (MHLW, 2013a). These data suggest that the services provide only for partial elderly care, meaning that the ratio of informal care increases as the designated degree of care rises. According to the 2012 Employment Status Survey report of the Ministry of Internal Affairs and Communications, the number of people whose employment has been affected by reasons associated with caring for elderly family members in the past five years is 480,007, with women accounting for about 80% at 380,009. Approximately 100,000 people a year have left work for reasons associated with care giving (Statistic Bureau, 2012).

With regard to the future of social care for older adults with mental health disorders, one of the most serious problems faced by Japan as a super-aged society is the employment of young people. It is estimated that half of the number of young employees are non-regular part-time workers. A weakening of the employment status and income of young people will result in increasing instability of the national insurance and national pension system. Unlike other developed countries, the hourly wage for part-time workers in Japan is about half that of full-time workers. The ratio of non-regular employee aged 25-34 was 10.7% in 1988, but increased to 27.5% in 2015 (Statistics Bureau, 2015c). These low-income young workers do not belong to any company-based insurance programmes and rely entirely on the National Health Insurance and National Pension systems, which are already facing financial crisis due to the shrinking number of contributors and increasing number of recipients. Poor employment opportunities for young people also discourage young couples from having children, resulting in a reduction of the birth rate.

Such a precarious situation for the younger generations has influenced the nature of the contemporary family structure (Allison, 2013). Vogel (2013), a psychotherapist and a researcher of Japanese families in transition for over 50 years, has documented that changes in Japanese society and economic uncertainty have fuelled a surge in new kinds of psychological disorders, including refusal to attend school, withdrawing from society (*hikikomori*), and sexless co-habitation. Prior to the Second World War, it was widely understood that the oldest son would inherit the family property and wealth, and assume the responsibility of supporting his ageing parents; in reality, however, his wife had the responsibility of taking care of older adults family members in Japan. If this notion of the eldest son receiving the family's inheritance in return for looking after his parents in their old age still exists among Japanese, then, as shown in the case of the family structure of the case of Mrs. H, above, the ability of unmarried sons or daughters to help ageing and older parents with disabilities seems to be greatly diminished, becoming a potential risk factor for the family and for society.

Conclusion

The Long-term Care Insurance system, a nationally mandated programme, changed the public's understanding of social care for older people. It turned what had previously been regarded as a service for the poor, into that of a social service available to all Japanese citizens. Considerable efforts have been made to provide a comprehensive service for older adults with mental health issues, however, the data suggests that the LTCI services still only provide partial care, therefore the economic burden on service users and their family largely remains.

Although universal coverage for pensions, health insurance, and the long-term care insurance has made it possible for Japanese citizens to live long healthy lives, Japan, as a 'super-aged' society, is confronted with an increasing number of socio-economic challenges. Both the fiscal viability of, and the ability to provide for an increasing demand on social care and welfare services in the future, depends on the fiscal and mental strength of the younger generation. The relationship between the sustainability of long-term care, and informal care which is mostly provided by family care givers, is perhaps the most important issue that needs to be addressed by both regional and national governments as Japan enters the welfare society of the future.

References

Allison, A. (2013). *Precarious Japan*. Durham and London: Duke University Press.

Cabinet Office. (2008). *Heisei 20nenban koureishakai hakusho (zentai ban)*. Retrieved from http://www8.cao.go.jp/kourei/whitepaper/w-2008/zenbun/html/s1-1-1-01.html.

Cabinet Office. (2012). *Heisei 24nenban koureishakai hakusho (zentai ban)*. Retrieved from http://www8.cao.go.jp/kourei/whitepaper/w-2012/zenbun/s1_2_1_01.html.

Cabinet Office. (2015a). *Nenji keizai zaisei houkoku*. Retrieved from http://www5.cao.go.jp/keizai3/2011/1221nk/n11_q/n11_q_1.html.

Campbell, J. C. (1993). *How policies change: The Japanese Government and aging society*. New Jersey: Princeton University Press.

Chibaken Minji Kyo (2015). *Minsei iin ni tsuite*. Retrieved from http://www.chiba-minkyo.or.jp/minsei-history.html.

Chuo Shakai Fukushi Singikai (1981). *Tomen no zaitaku rojin taisaku ni tsuite* (Iken gushin). Retrieved from http://www.ipss.go.jp/publication/j/shiryou/no.13/data/shiryou/syakaifukushi/178.pdf.

Chuo Shakai Hoshou Singikai Shougaisya Bukai Seishin Syougai Bunkai, 2002. *Houkokusyo; Kongono seishin hoken hukusi sisaku nituite*. Retrieved from http://www.mhlw. go.jp/shingi/2008/04/dl/s0411-7g.pdf.

Administration Bureau, Ministry of Internal Affair and Communication. (2015a). *Shouhi zei hou*. Retrieved from http://law.e-gov.go.jp/htmldata/S63/S63HO108.html.

Administration Bureau, Ministry of Internal Affair and Communication. (2015b).

Estévez-Abe, A. (2007). *Welfare and capitalism in postwar Japan*. Cambridge: Cambridge University Press.

Itou, H. (06/01/2013). *Togai shisetu nyukyosha 4 nen de 2.6 bai, 23 ku no kourei seikatuhogosha*. Ashahı shinbun. Retrieved from http://apital.asahi.com/article/news/2013010600001.html.

Kasza, G. (2006). *One world of welfare: Japan in comparative perspective*. Ithaca and London: Cornell University Press.

MacDonald, K. (2008). Agony of Eldercare; Two Japanese Woman Directors Study an Age-Old Problem. *Imaged Families Lived Families; Culture and Kinship in Contemporary Japan*. 51-73. State University of New York Press. Albany.

Ministry of Health and Welfare. (1989). *Koreisya hoken hukusi suisin 10 kanen keikaku. (Heisei 11 nendo made no 10 kanen keikaku)*. Retrieved from http://www.ipss.go.jp/publication/j/shiryou/no.13/data/shiryou/syakaifukushi/394.pdf.

Ministry of Health, Labor and Welfare. (1996). Patient Survey (*Kanjya chousa 1996*). Retrieved from http://www.e-stat.go.jp/SG1/estat/List.do?lid= 000001048340.

Ministry of Health, Labor and Welfare. (1999). Patient Survey (*Kanjya chousa*). Retrieved from http://www.e-stat.go.jp/SG1/estat/List.do?lid=0000010 48243.

Ministry of Health, Labor and Welfare. (2002). Patient Survey (*Kanjya chousa*). Retrieved from http://www.e-stat.go.jp/SG1/estat/List.do?lid=000001048 103.

Ministry of Health, Labor and Welfare. (2005a). Heisei 17 nendo no kaigo hoken seido kaikaku no kihonteki siten to omona naiyou. Retrieved from http://www.mhlw.go.jp/topics/kaigo/gaiyo/k2005_02.html.

Ministry of Health, Labor and Welfare. (2005b). Patient Survey (*Kanjya chousa*). Retrieved from http://www.e-stat.go.jp/SG1/estat/List.do?lid= 000001047095.

Ministry of Health, Labor and Welfare. (2007). *White paper (Heisei 19 nendo ban. Kosei rodo hakusyo)16-17*. Retrieved from http://www.mhlw.go.jp/wp/hakusyo/kousei/07/dl/0101.pdf.

Ministry of Health, Labor and Welfare. (2008). Patient Survey (*Kanjya chosa)*. Retrieved from http://www.e-stat.go.jp/SG1/estat/List.do?lid=000001 060228.

Ministry of Health, Labor and Welfare. (2011). Patient Survey (*Kanjya chousa*). Retrieved from http://www.e-stat.go.jp/SG1/estat/List.do? lid=000001103073.

Ministry of Health, Labor and Welfare. (2013a). Kokumin seikatu kiso chousa. Retrieved from http://www.mhlw.go.jp/toukei/list/20-21.html.

Ministry of Health, Labor and Welfare. (2013b). *White paper* (*Kosei rodo hakusyo)*. Retrieved from http://www.mhlw.go.jp/wp/hakusyo/kousei/13/dl/1-02-2.pdf.

Ministry of Health, Labor and Welfare. (2014). Demographic survey (*Jinko doutai toukei nenpyou*). Retrieved from http://www.mhlw.go.jp/toukei/saikin/hw/jinkou/suii10/dl/s03.pdf.

Ministry of Health, Labor and Welfare. (2015a). Dementia (*Ninchi syou*). Retrieved from http://www.mhlw.go.jp/kokoro/speciality/detail_recog. html.

Ministry of Health, Labor and Welfare. (2015b). *Procedures for using the system*. Retrieved from http://www.mhlw.go.jp/english/wp/wp-hw6/dl/10e.pdf.

Ministry of Health, Labor and Welfare. (2015c) *Yokaigo nintei.* Retrieved from http://www.mhlw.go.jp/stf/seisakunitsuite/bunya/hukushi_kaigo/kaigo_koureisha/nintei/.

Ministry of Health, Labor and Welfare. (2015d). *Health Care and Welfare Measures for Persons with Disabilities.* Retrieved from http://www.mhlw.go.jp/english/wp/wp-hw6/dl/09e.pdf.

Ministry of Justice. (2015a). The Constitution of Japan. Retrieved from http://www.japaneselawtranslation.go.jp/law/detail/?id=174&vm=04&re=01&new=1.

Ministry of Justice. (2015b). Act on Social Welfare for older adults. Retrieved from http://www.japaneselawtranslation.go.jp/law/detail/?id=2070&vm= 04&re=01.

Ministry of Justice. (2015c). Long-Term Care Insurance Act. Retrieved from http://www.japaneselawtranslation.go.jp/law/detail/?id=94&vm=04&re=01&new=1.

Ministry of Justice. (2015d). Services and Supports for Persons with Disabilities Act. Retrieved from http://www.japaneselawtranslation.go.jp/law/detail/?id=143.

National Institute of Population and Social Security Research. (2011). *Social Security in Japan (2011 edition).* Tokyo: NIPSSR.

National Institute of Population and Social Security Research. (2011). *Social Security in Japan (2014 edition).* Tokyo: NIPSSR.

Sabisu tuki Koureisha muke Jutaku. (2015). *Seido ni tuite.* Retrieved from http://www.satsuki-jutaku.jp/system.html.

Shougaisya no nitijou seikatu oyobi shakai seikatu wo sougouteki ni sien suru tameno houritsu. Retrieved from http://law.e-gov.go.jp/htmldata/H17/H17HO123.html.

Showa 63 Nendo Kosei Kagaku Tokubetu Kenkyu Jigyo. (2003). *Netakiri rojin no genjyou narabini syogaikoku to no hikakuni kansuru kenkyu.* Retrieved from http://www.ipss.go.jp/publication/j/shiryou/no.13/data/shiryou/syakaifukushi/388.pdf.Statistics Bureau. (2012). Syugyou kiso kouzou chousa. Retrieved from http://www.stat.go.jp/data/shugyou/2012/index.htm.

Statistics Bureau. (2015a). *Jinko suikei* (20 October 2014). Retrieved from http://www.stat.go.jp/data/jinsui/2014np/index.htm.

Statistics Bureau. (2015b). *Population Estimates* (March 2015). Retrieved from http://www.stat.go.jp/english/data/jinsui/tsuki/index.htm.

Statistics Bureau. (2015c).Labour force survey. Historical data 9. Retrieved from http://www.stat.go.jp/english/data/roudou/lngindex.htm.

Suga, Y.(1996). *Nihon no Home Help ni okeru Kaigo Hukusi Keiseisi.* Retrieved from http://www3.kumagaku.ac.jp/srs/pfd2/2-1/2-1-87.pdf.

Tsumura, A. (1973). Iryou no doukou. *Kikan Syakaihosyou Kenkyu (The Quarterly Social Security Research Journal), 9*(1), 36-47.

Vogel, S. and Vogel, S. (2013). *The Japanese family in transition: from the professional house wife ideal to the dilemmas of choice.* Plymouth: Rowman and Littlefield.

Zenkoku Caravan Meito Renraku Kyougikai. (2015). Ninchishou supporter no yousei jyoukyou, Retrieved from http://www.caravanmate.com/.

Zenkoku Minsei Iin Jidou Iin Rengoukai. (2015). *Minsei iin/jido iin no rekisi.* Retrieved from http://www2.shakyo.or.jp/zenminjiren/minsei_zidou_summary/history.html.

In: Ageing and Mental Health: Global Perspectives
Editors: Wendy Wen Li, Sherry M. Cummings et al.
ISBN: 978-1-63484-777-3

Chapter 9

AGEING AND MENTAL HEALTH IN PORTUGAL

Sofia von Humboldt[1,*] ***and Kassandra Jackson***[2]
[1]Instituto Universitário de Ciências Psicológicas, Sociais e da Vida, Lisboa, Portugal
[2]James Cook University, Queensland, Australia

ABSTRACT

Portugal is one of the most aged countries in the world and its population is continuing to age. The proportion of those over 65 constitutes an increasing proportion of the population, placing significant pressure on the Portuguese health care system to accommodate and respond to the needs of older Portuguese people. Risk of mental illness increases with age, and issues such as suicide and dementia are especially relevant to the older population. Most of Portugal's mental health care is provided generally, and specialised services aimed at older Portuguese are uncommon. Some programmes, such as the *National Health Plan*, do have specific objectives related to the improvement of older mental health outcomes, but these are not necessarily reflected in practice. The present chapter discusses the context of ageing in Portugal; the prevalence of mental illness among Portuguese and research into prevalence; mental health services and caregiving practices among the Portuguese; and the nature of mental health policy in Portugal. The chapter will conclude with a discussion of the gaps and future suggestions for research and policy.

Keywords: Portugal, mental health, caregiving, dementia, depression, suicide, policy

INTRODUCTION

Portugal is the seventh most aged country in the world (World Health Organization [WHO], 2011). Currently, there are nearly two million Portuguese aged 65 years and above (18% of the total population), which makes population ageing a pressing reality in Portugal. It is estimated that the total percentage of older Portuguese people (> 65 years old) in 2050 will

* Corresponding author. Email: sofia.humboldt@gmail.com.

be greater than 31% of the Portuguese population (Permanent Mission of Portugal to the United Nations, 2011; WHO, 2011). In recent years, along with the ageing of the population, there have been profound changes in the epidemiological pattern, socio-familial circumstances, and the profile of Portuguese older people (Permanent Mission of Portugal to the United Nations, 2011). Increased life expectancy is one of the major factors contributing to the ageing population, where life expectancy increased by 15.6 years between 1960 and 2009 (WHO, 2011). Furthermore, Portugal has one of the lowest fertility rates in all of Europe at 1.21 babies per woman. This means that each woman of childbearing age produces 1.21 children in their lifetime, which is not enough to replace themselves and their partner (WHO, 2011). The ageing population has become a strategic challenge for the central and local health and social care policies in Portugal[1]. It is anticipated that the psychogeriatric needs of the older population will increase in the near future, placing more pressure on the health care system to implement adequate mental health services for older Portuguese.

This chapter will discuss the context of ageing in Portugal and the prevalence information of mental illness among the elderly. The nature of mental health services and caregiving will then be explored, followed by the political context of mental health in Portugal. Finally, the gaps in mental health identification and treatment among the elderly in Portugal will be identified, and recommendations will be made for future changes.

THE CONTEXT OF AGEING AND MENTAL HEALTH IN PORTUGAL

Existing literature has highlighted that the prevalence of mental health problems in Portugal could be higher than in other European countries, while the most vulnerable groups (the aged, women, and the poor) seemed to exhibit a further increased risk of mental illness (European Opinion Research Group [EORG], 2003; Gusmão, Xavier, Heitor, Bento and Almeida, 2005; Kovess-Masféty et al., 2006; Xavier et al., 2013). In 2002, more than a third of adults aged over 65 years in Portugal were diagnosed with mental health problems, namely depression and dementia (EORG, 2003; Wittchen and Jacobi, 2005).

Demographic changes in Portugal seem to have followed global trends towards ageing. Portuguese society has shifted from a demographically young welfare country to an ageing society. The increased percentage of people 65 years and older and the decreased percentage younger than 15 years has resulted in a double ageing effect (Caldas de Almeida, Xavier and Mateus, 2008; EORG, 2003). This ageing has been followed by a growth in the prevalence of mental illness. Hence, Portugal is currently dealing with increasing psychogeriatric needs among the older population, and is lacking the services to deliver them. Furthermore, this demographic transition has resulted in an increased government budget deficit and a rise in unemployment levels, which has a negative impact on psychiatric morbidity in old age (Caldas de Almeida et al., 2008; European Research Infrastructure Consortium, 2011).

Approximately 30% of the older population in Portugal lives in a state of poverty, although this number has been somewhat reduced in recent years (Caldas de Almeida et al., 2008; Centro de Estudos e Desenvolvimento Regional e Urbano and Boston Consulting

[1] Central government and local government in Portugal articulate a general network of health services, composed of district hospitals and local community health assistance centres.

Group, 2008). In addition, there is concern over regional disparities, particularly between urban-coastal and rural-interior regions. The latter have the highest poverty rates, the worst mental health conditions, and have been faced with high population ageing associated with a large exodus of young and working age people. Indeed, the migration of the population from the interior to the coastal cities has been progressively increasing in the last two decades.

The waves of migration to Portugal have been diverse in terms of socio-economic status and cultural and ethnic background, and large suburban areas were built to hold the influx of internal and external immigrants (Caldas de Almeida et al., 2008). Cultural, national, and ethnic differences may influence the perceptions of ageing (Barak, 2009; Löckenhoff, et al., 2009); however, diverse perceptions of ageing have produced little impact in the current demographic trends.

Currently, there are 394,496 foreigners living in Portugal (3.7% of overall population) (Instituto Nacional de Estatística, 2011). Immigration to Portugal is mainly from Brazil, Central and Eastern Europe, and Africa. Several foreign communities currently reside in Portugal, the most representative older groups being from Brazil, Portuguese-speaking African countries, Germany and the United Kingdom. Yet, little is known about these older inhabitants' mental condition (von Humboldt, Leal and Pimenta, 2014). In line with these demographic changes, the Portuguese mental health care system is still struggling to address some of the specific challenges presented by recent legal and illegal immigration (Caldas de Almeida et al., 2008). Urbanisation and migration has resulted in some difficulties in accessing mental health services for older people, particularly those living in rural areas. Likewise, the rapid expansion of the suburban neighborhoods has changed the traditional family and social networks, thus increasing the sense of isolation, low accessibility, and non-integration for Portuguese older adults with mental health conditions (Caldas de Almeida et al., 2008).

Equity and accessibility of mental health care in Portugal is a result of perceived health needs of the older population and lifestyle, economic, and social factors, such as income, urbanisation, migration, living conditions and unemployment (Caldas de Almeida et al., 2008; Centro de Estudos e Desenvolvimento Regional e Urbano and Boston Consulting Group, 2008; Santana, 2000). The ageing phenomenon, reduced population density of the inland regions, urban concentration along the coast, the growth of functional dependency, and the diversity of health care needs have directly influenced mental health service access and usage among older populations. Existing mental health plans and legislation are aimed at assuring equity in access to mental health care in old age, decentralising services, increasing proximity care, promoting mental health in old age, preventing depression and suicide, and promoting and protecting human rights (WHO, 2011). While mental health care is considered a right and is guaranteed to all older adults by law in Portugal, limits imposed by financial, human, and technical resources reduce the real impact of the legislation. Indeed, accessibility to mental health care is not the same in all geographical areas and for all groups of the population. Age is one of the most important factors that can influence usage associated with location, and older people are at a disadvantage with respect to the delivery of mental health care (Santana, 2000). Additionally, in rural areas where population ageing is more noticeable, there is a higher percentage of older people living alone and a less diversified network of mental health care services (Santana, 2000).

Mental illness, like ageing, carries the meaning that society places on it. Mental health in old age still carries myths, prejudices, and stereotypes, despite the growing investment in related research and treatment. In Portugal, stigma and discrimination related to mental disorders are associated with suffering, disability, and economic waste. Therefore, older Portuguese people with mental disorders carry a double burden when it comes to stereotyping and prejudice which merits special attention (Caldas de Almeida, 2009; Santana, 2000; WHO, 2008). Policies for fighting stigma, discrimination, and social exclusion, currently support older adults at social risk and assess the impact of social policies in mental health. Further social protection, social inclusion, and integration are necessary to break the cycle of discrimination based on mental health problems and age, and also to bring forward comprehensive care for older people with mental health problems (Santana, 2000; WHO, 2008).

THE PREVALENCE OF OLDER PORTUGUESE ADULTS' MENTAL HEALTH DISORDERS

There is a lack of national research in Portugal that investigates mental illness in the older population. Among those studies that have been conducted, the primary focus has been on depression, dementia, and suicide. As a result, little is known about other mental health conditions in later life in Portugal (von Humboldt, Leal and Pimenta, 2012). The present section discusses the prevalence of depression, anxiety, dementia, suicide, and substance abuse among older Portuguese.

Depression and Anxiety

According to the National Health Survey (2005/2006), 27.6% of the general Portuguese population present with symptoms of depression or anxiety. Although ageing does not necessarily lead to an increase of depressive disorders, recent studies have suggested that depression is the most common mental health problem experienced by older adults in Portugal. Despite this, reported prevalence of depression among older adults in literature has been inconsistent (e.g., Almeida and Quintão, 2012; Oliveira Santos, Cruvinel and Neri 2006). According to the Instituto Nacional de Estatística, between 2005 and 2006, 183,428 adults aged 65 or over showed symptoms of depression (Minghelli, Tomé, Nunes, Neves and Simões, 2013). In comparison, some studies have suggested that depression affects between 6% and 10% of the population aged 65 or over (Frade, Barbosa, Cardoso and Nunes, 2015; Gusmão et al., 2005; Xavier, Ferraz and Trendi, 2001). Passos and his colleagues (2012) concluded that 36% of a sample comprising 75 adults aged 65 or over and with mental illness were diagnosed with depression. In the same sample, bipolar disorder was found to be the third most common mental health condition (12%) and situational depression one of the fourth most common mental health conditions (5.3%). Moreover, Ponte, Almeida and Fernandes (2014) concluded that of a sample comprising 75 adults aged 65 or over in gerontopsychiatry consultations at a hospital in Porto, 66.7% presented with severe depression and suicidal ideation. Evidently, research indicating the actual rates of depression and anxiety in the older population is conflicting, suggesting a need for further research in this area.

Age is considered a risk factor for the onset of depressive symptoms in Portugal. Pimenel, Afonso, and Pereira (2012) investigated depression prevalence among 117 individuals over the age of 65, and results suggested that those over 75 years old showed higher levels of depression than those younger than that age. Furthermore, in a review of studies investigating depression among older people living in the community compared to those in care institutions, it was found that 14% of older adults living in the community showed, and73% of institutionalised older adults (Pimentel et al., 2012).

Research has suggested that the prevalence of depression among older Portuguese may be underestimated (Caldas de Almeida et al., 2008; Passos et al., 2012; Pimentel et al. 2012). A number of factors contribute to this underestimation. Firstly, as older adults with clinically significant depressive symptoms do not often meet the DSM-IV criteria for depression, health care professionals may identify depressive symptoms as a standard response to other severe conditions, such as dementia, or even to the social and financial adversities that often go hand-in-hand with ageing (Veríssimo, 2006). Secondly, under-diagnosis of depression may be related to active denial by older patients (Oliveira et al., 2006). Thirdly, assessment and diagnosis of elderly depression in Portugal is underachieved by health care services, since they may fail to see when older people present with depression (Garcia et al., 2006, Oliveira et al., 2006).

There is insufficient recent research concerning the prevalence of anxiety in late adulthood in Portugal. Moreover, until the last decade, anxiety disorders were still a relatively unidentified mental health issue among older adults (Passos et al., 2012; Wetherell, Lenze and Stanley, 2005). Passos and his colleagues (2012) investigated anxiety prevalence among 75 adults over the age of 65 in the North of Portugal. Among those who participated, 4% were diagnosed with anxiety. More recently, Minghelli and her colleagues (2013) compared a sample of sedentary and active adults aged 65 and above. These authors found that 16.7% of the sedentary older adults and 5.6% of the active older adults showed symptoms of anxiety. This suggests that there may be a relationship between level of activity and anxiety among older adults. The nature of anxiety in older adulthood in Portugal is uncertain, hindering proper assessment and intervention (Bryant, Jackson and Ames, 2008; Minghelli et al., 2013).

The lack of literature investigating how depression and anxiety presents among older Portuguese adults, as well as their prevalence, uncovers a relevant gap in understanding. Further research in this area may improve the effectiveness of interventions and treatment for affected older Portuguese.

Dementia

Dementia is a comprehensive term for over one hundred diseases affecting cognitive function. Among the most common forms of dementia are Alzheimer's disease, vascular dementia, dementia with Lewy bodies, and fronto-temporal dementia. Dementia usually implies deficits to cognitive abilities, most often memory decline, behavioural disorders, and loss of the person's autonomy (Caltagirone, Perri, Carlesimo and Fadda, 2001; von Humboldt and Leal, 2012; Washburn and von Humboldt, 2013).

Despite worldwide recognition of the burden of dementia, no epidemiological data is yet available in Portugal (Nunes et al., 2010). The ageing of Portugal's population has led to an increased number of older adults with dementia (Passos et al., 2012). In a study comprising one sample from a rural Portuguese community and one from an urban Portuguese community involving 1049 adults aged 55 to 79 years, dementia was present in 2.7% of participants. Additionally, it was higher in rural (16.8%) than in urban (12%) populations (Nunes et al., 2010). In another study investigating the needs of older people with mental health problems, 75 older adults were recruited from the National Health Service in the Inpatient and Outpatient Department of Psychiatry and Mental Health at a Health Unit in Northern Portugal. Of those aged 65 years and above, 29.3% suffered from dementia (Passos et al., 2012).

It is difficult to distinguish dementia from the common effects of ageing on cognitive function. Older adults may present with a decline in cognitive functioning that can appear to be dementia, but actually be related to other age factors such as sensory decline or health deterioration. Indeed, it is estimated that up to 10% of patients aged 65 years and above are misdiagnosed by general practitioners and family doctors to have dementia, when in fact they have an illness with similar symptoms, such as depression, delirium, a cerebral tumour, hypothyroidism, folic acid deficiency or renal failure. Accordingly, dementia assessment should investigate a wide range of factors that may influence older patients' conditions (Brayne, Fox and Boustani, 2007; Gelder, Mayou and Geddes, 2006).

Suicide

Suicide is a serious public health problem among older adults in Portugal (Caldas de Almeida et al., 2008). As with many countries, the suicide rate in Portugal increases with age. Correspondingly, the highest suicide rate is in the over 50 age group, at 13 suicides per 100,000 people (Sampaio and Telles-Correia, 2013). Comparatively, suicide rates in 2009 were at 9.64 per 100,000 for the general population in Portugal. Between 1980 and 2009, deaths by suicide increased by 30% (Caldas de Almeida et al., 2008). Mental health conditions including major depression, severe anxiety, schizophrenia, borderline personality disorders and alcohol abuse are strongly associated with suicide in old age (Minayo and Cavalcante, 2010; Sampaio and Telles-Correia, 2013).

Among the older population, the highest suicide rates were found in males aged 75 years and above (60 per 100,000). The highest suicide rate for females was also in the 75 years and over age group at 10.7 per 100,000 (Sociedade Portuguesa de Suicidologia, 2009). Although males are already more likely to commit suicide, the suicide rate for men seems to be increasing, while for the women aged 65 years and above, the figure is decreasing (Caldas de Almeida et al., 2008).

Older adults seem to prepare their suicide cautiously and the methods are more lethal in order to increase their efficacy (Quintão, Costa, Alves and Gusmão, 2013). The most used lethal methods by older Portuguese adults were hanging (50.0%), ingesting of poison (13.68%) and intentional drowning (8.73%) (Quintão et al., 2013). The absence of a prevention programme specifically catering to older adults with mental health disorders currently hampers the prevention of this public health problem.

Substance Abuse

The number of European older people with substance use problems or requiring treatment for a substance use disorder is estimated to more than double between 2001 and 2020. Between 2002 and 2005, the proportion of reported patients aged 40 or over being treated for opiate problems more than doubled (from 8.6% to 17.6%) (General-Directorate for Intervention on Addictive Behaviours and Dependencies [SICAD], 2014). Current evidence in relation to Portuguese older adults is limited mainly to alcohol abuse, making it difficult to estimate the precise extent and implications of substance use and dependence, such as illicit and prescription drugs (SICAD, 2014). In a study conducted in 2012 in the Portuguese general population, cannabis, ecstasy and cocaine were the illicit substances preferably used by the Portuguese with lifetime prevalence (at least one use experience) respectively of 9.4%, 1.3% and 1.2%. Between 2007 and 2012, a decrease in lifetime prevalence was verified for almost all drugs in the Portuguese population (of any illicit drug from 12% to 9.5%) and recent use (of any illicit drug from 3.7% to 2.7%) as well as decrease in continuity rates of use (of any illicit drug from 31% to 28%) (SICAD, 2014). Portuguese legislation has decriminalised the use of drugs, with the primary objective being to reduce drug use and to safeguard the needs of individuals at preventive, health and therapeutic levels. For this objective, the Commissions for the Dissuasion of Drug Use (CDT) were created in each capital district to develop work with the vulnerable groups of the population in close proximity, such as older adults, in the mediation between situations of use and the application of administrative sanctions (SICAD, 2014).

Alcohol related issues are integrated within the context of mental health and are included in the Portuguese general health system (Jané-Llopis and Anderson, 2006). This is because Portugal is among the countries with the highest alcohol per person consumption in the world (9.38 liters in 2003) (Caldas et al., 2008). Passos and his colleagues (2012) investigated alcohol dependence among 75 individuals aged over 65 who had been diagnosed with a mental illness. This study found that alcohol dependence was one of the most common mental health conditions in this population, with 5.3% of participants reportedly dependant on alcohol. Substance abuse can have a strong effect on concentration, attention, and cognition (Goudie, 2002), and may even trigger schizophrenia in older adults. Substance abuse, including alcohol dependence, is still an under-identified public health problem of reasonable proportions in Portugal. The symptoms of substance abuse may also hamper the diagnosis and treatment of other mental health conditions among older people (Menninger, 2002).

Mental Health Services for Older Portuguese Adults

Older adults share mental health services with the rest of the population, making it difficult to analyse specialised services for this age group. These services include mental hospitals and community based psychiatric inpatient and outpatient units in general hospitals. Moreover, the public national healthcare system covers mental health treatment, such as psychotherapy or psychotropic medication for older adults with mental conditions (EORG, 2003).

The prevalence of individuals with mental health conditions is 16.07%, yet only 1.7% of older Portuguese with mental health problems have access to specialised mental health services (Caldas de Almeida et al., 2008). Twenty-four per cent of older patients are admitted for inpatient mental health hospitalisation and 71% of older patients with mental health problems receive outpatient treatment in general hospitals (Caldas de Almeida, 2009). The number of older people using mental health services is particularly low (17% of the older population), compared to what could be expected. Such services are often used only by those with severe mental illness (Xavier et al., 2013).

The majority of mental health services are concentrated in Lisbon, Porto and Coimbra. Services created in the rest of the country are only operated partially and some units are not operational due to a lack of staff (Caldas de Almeida et al., 2008). Additionally, regional discrepancies are most noticeable for groups that show the highest need for health care in Portugal, such as older adults. Because of physical limitations due to age and scarcity of services in rural areas, older individuals living in these areas have limited access to health care. In fact, age is one of the most significant variables that can influence access to services in different areas (Santana, 2000).

In 2013 in the general population, admissions to community based psychiatric inpatient units in general and mental hospitals across the country were at 194 people per 100,000 (Xavier et al., 2013). In comparison, the combined number of psychiatric beds per 100,000 general population available in mental hospitals, community psychiatric inpatient units, and units in district general hospitals, was only 27 (Xavier et al., 2013). However, in the case of Portugal, fewer beds are a result of deinstitutionalisation and not a lack of service infrastructure. The loss of mental hospital beds has been substituted with the presence of small-scale, local community services such as religious residential facilities, which serve older adults with lack of autonomy and mental health problems (Jané-Llopis and Anderson, 2006; WHO, 2008).

The rate of visits to mental health outpatient facilities in 2005 was 5323 people per 100,000 of the general population. Outpatient health care is offered in mental hospitals, district general hospitals, or in purpose-built units, but seldom in community settings. Portuguese mental health policy also warrants access to crisis care 24 hours a day and access to home treatment for people with mental disorders. These patients also have access to rehabilitation services and community residential health facilities. However, there are only 2.2 beds in community residential health facilities per 100,000 general population and 34 beds in facilities that are not aimed at health care per 100,000 general population (Xavier et al., 2013; WHO, 2008).

In Portugal, the basis of the health care system is the Social Security System. This covers most mental health care costs including treatment in mental hospitals, inpatient units, community-based psychiatric care, and outpatient unit costs in district general hospitals. All Portuguese residents, regardless of citizenship status, are eligible for the same Social Security System benefits and have access to any of these mental health services (Jané-Llopis and Anderson, 2006).

Portuguese mental health care is not limited to policy mandated services. There are 62 non-governmental organisations (NGOs) working in mental health among the elderly which provide supported employment, social support, counselling, social skills training, and leisure and occupational activities for older people with mental health problems. Fifty-four NGO community services, supporting 992 people with mental health conditions, are partly funded by the government. Additionally, the government funds social occupational units, supported residences, and companies that employ older people with mental health problems (Caldas de Almeida et al., 2008; Jané-Llopis and Anderson, 2006).

The cost of psychotropic medication for use in mental health hospitals is funded by the Portuguese Social Security System which covers approximately 80% (WHO, 2008). Medication is available free of charge or fully reimbursed for older people with severe mental health problems, especially in hospital settings. Psychotherapy is supported at least 80% by public funds but is not available at all hospitals or in community services. Access and reimbursement to psychotherapy by older adults is strictly controlled in Portugal and is not always available, especially in primary care. Hence, the probability of receiving psychotherapy for mental health issues decreases for older service users (WHO, 2008).

Portuguese mental health services also lack specialised professionals. Most mental health services rely on a small number of psychologists, nurses, social workers, occupational therapists, and other non-medical professionals. The number of psychiatrists, psychologists, and nurses per 100,000 in the general population, is 6.7, 2.3, and 13.2 respectively (Caldas de Almeida et al., 2008). In mental health practices with older adults, professionals most commonly assess cognitive functions, despite acknowledging the diverse and influential factors affecting the well-being and mental health of these patients. Portuguese mental health policy expects general practitioners (GPs) or family doctors to identify, diagnose and treat older adults. This means GPs or family doctors also play a major role in identifying, diagnosing, and treating severe mental disorders. Treatment is not always expected to be the responsibility of the relevant specialists, specifically, geriatric psychiatrists. Frequently and except for the treatment of severe mental disorders that may require hospitalisation, the role of Portuguese family doctors seems to extend beyond the responsibilities that are specified in policy guidance and may involve psychiatric interventions. This is possibly explicated by a blend of expectations, tradition, ethics, and acceptance (WHO, 2008). Anderson (2007) suggested that older adults are at a disadvantage with respect to the delivery of mental health services in comparison with the rest of the population, despite having the same and often greater needs. In relation to this, Portugal offers more specialised training to psychiatrists for treating children than for older people, which again reflects a bias against older adults (WHO, 2008).

Existing results from the *National Mental Health Plan Report* show that Portuguese mental health services suffer from serious deficiencies in terms of impartiality, availability, and quality of care (Xavier et al., 2013). Local mental health services are limited to hospitalisation, outpatient consultations, and day hospital. There are no community mental healthcare services that perform integrated case management, crisis intervention or programmes involving families, adding to the lack of efficacy of Portuguese care services. In this context, adopting an approach addressing some of the aspects discussed above could provide more specified and directed interventions for older adults. Given the ageing population in Portugal, these issues are increasingly important to ensure positive outcomes for the older Portuguese population and Portuguese society as a whole.

To combat social exclusion among vulnerable groups in Portugal such as older adults and in particular, women, the Fe–Formemprego was created in 2002. The Fe-Formemprego is a government initiative which targets people with a mental illness who are struggling with social and professional integration. The programme is aimed at developing the potential of older people with mental conditions and supporting professional integration, taking into account their individual abilities and life projects. To achieve this, the programme provides flexible orientation and training, as well as support in finding an appropriate workplace which reflects the skills and needs of each individual (Jané-Llopis and Anderson, 2006).

Informal Caregiving and Social Support

The quality of social support has direct positive effects on older adults' health and can buffer or reduce some of the health-related effects of ageing (Cornwell, Schumm, Laumann, Kim and Kim, 2014). In fact, many older individuals with mental health needs receive help from family, friends, and social or religious institutions. In 2012, it was estimated that 1.1% of older Portuguese adults aged 65 years and over receive some type of caregiving support. Of this group, 0.9% of individuals receive long-term support in institutions whilst 0.1% received caregiving support at home. From these, 63% was performed by their families and 13% by institutional caregivers working in the community (Unidade de Missão dos Cuidados Continuados Integrados, 2012).

Historically, Portuguese culture has been strongly family-oriented, with family members traditionally taking responsibility for caregiving of the elderly. As a result of demographic and socio-economic shifts, such as lower fertility rates, smaller households, and urbanisation, people are becoming less likely to take up the role of carer for their aged family members. Research investigating the socio-economic antecedents of caregiving demonstrates that older Portuguese adults and families from lower socio-economic strata are more likely to end up in informal caregiving roles. Individuals from higher socio-economic classes have, and often take advantage of, greater financial flexibility to contract out all or some of their care work. Although the majority of older adults are still reliant on informal care, informal care is converging with formal care in home and community settings (Wall, Aboim, Cunha and Vasconcelos, 2001).

Research has suggested that women are more likely to act as caregivers. Sequeira (2013) investigated Portuguese caregiving in a study comprising 184 Portuguese caregivers over 40 years of age, of which 101 cared for dependent people without cognitive impairment and 83 cared for people with dementia. Most caregivers were women (87%) and most were married (78.8%). Additionally, most caregivers were spouses or daughters (75.5%). In another similar study, Alves and his colleagues (2015) found that informal caregivers had an average age of 52.08 years, were mainly women (90.0%), and were married/partnered (75.0%). As women are more likely to act as caregivers, their increased presence in the labour force reduces their availability for caregiving, further reducing the number of available informal carers and putting pressure on health care services. These social and demographic changes may contribute to the decrease in traditional resilience of family networks as the primary welfare providers for older adults (Melchiorre et al., 2013).

Melchiorre and her colleagues (2013) conducted a study investigating levels of social support among 4,467 individuals aged 60-84 in seven countries across Europe. Of these, Portugal was reported to have the lowest score on social support compared with those of other European countries. In this study, lower levels of social support were related to older age and abuse, particularly psychological abuse. Portuguese older people may therefore receive comparatively less social support, especially those who are older and have experienced psychological abuse.

Insufficient social support may play a role in mediating the mental health of older Portuguese adults. Paúl and her colleagues (2003) conducted a study investigating the psychosocial profile of 234 independent, older Portuguese people drawn from rural and urban Portuguese settings. They concluded that both groups experienced some level of loneliness, suggesting that neither living in a rural nor urban setting ensures that older people will receive social support (Paúl, Fonseca, Martin and Amado, 2003). Another study involving the 25 EU member states, with the exception of the UK, conducted 72 qualitative interviews investigating risk factors for social exclusion among older adults. The findings suggested that living in rural areas was the main risk factor for social exclusion among older adults in Portugal due to a lack of access to social services (Hoff, 2008). This absence of social support may have severe effects on the well-being and mental health of older Portuguese adults with low income and who experience loneliness, which can lead to mental health problems and early institutionalisation. It must be noted that social isolation could be both a symptom and a cause of mental health problems (Melchiorre et al., 2013). Hoff (2008) indicated that needing care was one of the key risk factors for social exclusion in Portugal. Therefore, those older Portuguese who need care for a disability, dementia, or poor health may be even more likely to suffer social exclusion. To support older adults in obtaining care, a free telephone help line (Elderly Citizens Line) was established to make it easier to access available support services and establish links with caregivers (Hoff, 2008).

The effects of caring may have a negative impact on caregivers' lives in a variety of ways. Caregivers are at risk emotionally and physically, especially for stress-related illnesses. Piercy and colleagues (2012) conducted a study investigating depression among 256 carers of older people. They found that caregivers of older people with dementia were more depressed than those caring for someone with physical health problems (Piercy et al., 2012). This highlights the importance of adequate support systems for carers of older people suffering a mental illness.

Demographic characteristics, including sex and relationship to the care recipient may also be an important moderator of the impact of caregiving on mental health. Indeed, women, and particularly spouses and daughters take on more caregiving tasks, report more care recipient problems and experience more distress due to caregiving than male caregivers (Pinqüart and Sörensen, 2003, 2005). Legal and ethical issues may put further strain on the caregiving relationship, especially when that relationship is between family members. For example, confidentiality (such as when seeking consent to mental health treatment) and financial management may be contentious topics, increasing the stress experienced by the carer (Ryan and Coughlan, 2013). To address the best interests of older Portuguese adults and their caregivers, a full range of local and specialist services which support treatment and intervention are necessary, and cooperation between families, care settings, services, and institutional staff must be prioritised.

THE POLICY CONTEXT FOR OLDER ADULTS WITH MENTAL HEALTH ISSUES IN PORTUGAL

Portuguese mental health policy incorporates prevention, promotion and treatment of mental conditions, and psychosocial reintegration (Santos, 2006). Mental health in old age was selected as a main concern under the framework of the *National Health Plan* for 2004-2010 and 2008-2016. Portugal was one of the first European countries to institute a law acknowledging and attending to mental health in 1963, and mental health continues to be a priority in the national health context. Portuguese legislation covers aspects of mental health such as mental health centres, social psychiatry, and integration of mental health in primary care. In 1998, further additions to the Health Law 36/98[2] introduced the principles of mental health policy, organisation of services, and protection of human rights of people with mental disorders. In the same year, the law 407/98[3] sustained by the European Union Horizon 2020 reinforced the development of psychosocial rehabilitation services (Caldas de Almeida et al., 2008). The Portuguese mental health policy was later delineated in the Health Strategy for 2002 and in the Portuguese National Health Plan for 2004-2010 and involved health, social security, employment and social integration (Santos, 2006).

Furthermore, the Health Strategy for 2002 and the Portuguese *National Health Plan* for 2008-2016 addressed some central issues concerning the older population. The Health Strategy and National Health Plan intend to improve the diagnosis of health needs, provide enhanced care to older people by local communities and families, and improve rehabilitation and health care. They also aim to improve the training of gerontology and geriatric care professionals, assist with the implementation of local networks of integrated home care, and aid with the improvement of older adults' quality of life (Santana, 2000; Xavier et al., 2013). Since its implementation, the *National Health Plan* has been progressively revised to mirror societal changes and the current challenges of mental health. Currently the Portuguese *National Health Plan* for 2008-2016 addresses some central issues that affect the older population: amplification of mental health services; improvement of community mental health services; formation of a national network of psychosocial rehabilitation facilities; and implementation of prevention and promotion programmes, in particular in the areas of depression, suicide and alcohol. An example of this was the creation of a national programme on the prevention of depression: the European Alliance Against Depression (Jané-Llopis and Anderson, 2006).

Since 1998, there has been a continuous integration of social support for Portuguese individuals with mental health conditions in situations of considerable dependency (physical, mental, social) under the National Integrated Continuous Care Network which is funded by social security (Jané-Llopis and Anderson, 2006). The National Integrated Continuous Care Network provides specialised continuous care in terms of mental health for older adults in their communities, whilst stimulating social integration, as opposed to limiting them to mental health institutions (Caldas de Almeida et al., 2008).

---

[2] Mental health legislation (Law no. 36/98) (*in Portuguese*): http://dre.pt/application/dir/pdf1s/1998/07/169A00/35443550.pdf.

[3] Mental health legislation (Law no. 407/98) (*in Portuguese*): http://www4.seg-social.pt/documents/10152/35243/Desp_C_407_98.

In the last two decades, Portuguese policies have given priority to developing community services and downsising large mental hospitals. As an example, it is projected that by 2016, all local mental health services will be assisted by specialised mental health departments in general hospitals (Caldas de Almeida, 2009). Proactive policies for health promotion and disease prevention still need to be further developed. Since the 1990s, long-term public hospital beds and community primary health services have been continuously reduced; and concurrently, social private institutions, such as religious ones, have increased their shared responsibility concerning the older population (WHO, 2008). Adjusting mental health care to older adults' needs may decrease costs at the hospital level and consolidate the many levels of health care.

Since 2005, existing policies have been amended and new policies have been introduced to improve how mental health is addressed in Portugal. Despite this, variables impacting older adults' mental health such as diet, housing, and occupational health risks, are still insufficiently addressed in the health and welfare policies (Santana, 2000; WHO, 2008). Other challenges, such as the lack of adequate workforce, quality assurance, administrative organisation, information technology systems, partnerships, and funding, need to be further addressed when developing community-based mental services for older adults.

Treatment guidelines for the main mental health conditions such as dementia, mood disorders, psychotic conditions, substance abuse and suicide, do exist in general. For example, legislation specifies the role of GPs in identifying and treating people with common but not severe and permanent mental health problems. These are valuable in ensuring that professionals provide high-quality, up-to-date, evidence-based health care and that older adults that use health care services recognise what standards of care should be available for them (WHO, 2008). Despite this, guaranteeing that health professionals act in accordance with these guidelines has been a continuous challenge. Existing guidelines indicate that older adults with diagnosed severe mental health conditions are to be treated by mental health professionals in the general hospital or the community health centre. Additionally, guidelines for the coordination between the GPs and the mental health professionals are also available for the older population (WHO, 2008).

Although older Portuguese adults are entitled to the right of mental health protection, current human, technological and financial means constrain the current coverage of legislation and government policies. Older adults need health assistance more often, for longer periods and recurrently with a higher cost, compared to other age groups. Additionally, needs and access to services by older adults are not equally met in various geographical areas. Increased longevity and the number of older adults have led to an upsurge of health care costs with the older population. However, health care has not been adequately supported by objective mental health policy measures that reflect current needs. This is especially noticeable in rural areas where an increasing number of older adults are living alone and with less differentiated health care services. In such rural settings, difficulties in getting a medical appointment with a specialised mental health professional may restrict older adults' utilisation patterns and frequency (Santana, 2000).

Perceived discrimination may have a damaging impact on the health of older adults, contributing to increased illness and social isolation. The stigma attached to having a mental illness and being aged has an unbalanced effect on those regarded as both (Ryan and Coughlan, 2013). Presently, there are no policies that attempt to address this subject, allowing the continuation of institutionalised discrimination and ageism, with future negative impact on funding, training, service provision, research and collaboration with older adults and their families (Ryan and Coughlan, 2013). Involvement by governments is thus critical to stop discrimination and stigma and to improve social inclusion (WHO, 2008).

In summary, there is a pressing need for Portuguese health policies to define concrete objectives, approaches, and programmes which specifically address the needs of older adults with mental illness. They should further promote equal mental health treatment and a higher quality of life for older adults with diverse lifestyle, social, economic and geographical characteristics.

Gaps and Recommendations Concerning Portuguese Mental Health Care

Presently, not enough is known about the mental health problems of the elderly in Portugal. A lack of research, complications regarding diagnosis, and stereotypes surrounding ageing and mental health suggest a need for increased education regarding elderly mental illness. Correspondingly, services for older mental illness sufferers are limited, with older sufferers often forced to use generalised services and only infrequently accessing services specifically for older Portuguese (Caldas de Almeida, 2009; WHO, 2008). Following are a number of recommendations to improve the education and services available to elderly Portuguese with mental illness.

Education and Research

There are a number of difficulties associated with identifying mental health disorders in the elderly. Enduring and pressing mental health problems among older Portuguese adults such as depression, anxiety, dementia, alcohol abuse, and suicide, need to be specifically addressed (Caldas de Almeida, 2009). Increased education and research into the nature and presence of mental illness in the older population could serve to improve assessment and diagnosis. Presently, mental health problems may be underdiagnosed, and thus, not suitably addressed as a consequence of the belief that these problems are a normal component of the ageing process (WHO, 2008). Cognitive assessment is frequently used in routine clinical settings, although it is an insufficient indicator of the mental health of older adults since it does not consider, for example, their degree of adaptive functioning and psychological assessment. Due to the multifaceted interaction of psychological, physical, and social variables in older Portuguese adults, a multidisciplinary assessment and intervention is needed (WHO, 2008). This will ensure a comprehensive approach to mental health care with older adults. Indeed, the shortage and poor administrative organisation of mental health teams delivering multidisciplinary care to older adults is a critical gap, and improved education and research in this area will serve to address it.

Among the Portuguese population, ageism is a prevalent issue. Not only are older Portuguese discriminated against, but additional support and attention is paid only to the younger population, creating a kind of double discrimination (Caldas de Almeida, 2009; Santana, 2000; WHO, 2008). To further support older Portuguese suffering mental illness, it is necessary to provide education which discourages stigma surrounding old age and mental health, and aims to reduce the bias inherent in the health care system. Government policy and community initiatives should encourage interaction between older Portuguese with mental illness and the general population. This would serve to reduce social exclusion in this group while helping to break down barriers and reduce the prevalence of stereotypes. Furthermore, policy should encourage services to attend to older Portuguese suffering mental illness, who often require a greater level of assistance than the general population.

Service Provision

Presently, there are a number of areas in which elderly mental health care services could be improved. Services and health care providers currently under diagnose dementia due to it sharing common symptoms with other mental illnesses. Furthermore, common signs of ageing may be misdiagnosed as dementia, leading to inappropriate health care (WHO, 2008). To reduce misdiagnosis of mental illness among the older population, it would be beneficial to implement timely identification of mental health conditions through collaborative primary health care services. It would also be valuable to introduce services which primarily target comorbidity among older adults, in order to attend to the specific needs of that population (Jané-Llopis and Anderson, 2006; WHO, 2008).

Older adult mental health care would also benefit from a multidisciplinary approach. Considering the many common health problems in addition to mental illness within this population, it would be valuable to approach health care holistically. This could be achieved by ensuring that health care providers from many disciplines working with older individuals are equipped to communicate and work together to achieve positive health outcomes (Jané-Llopis and Anderson, 2006; WHO, 2008). Furthermore, developing a patient-centred approach which promotes general wellbeing for older people, their families, and their caregivers may serve to empower them throughout the treatment process. Engaging family and patients in planning and developing mental health services, as well as during treatment, will enable closer communication between service providers and their clients (WHO, 2008; Xavier et al., 2013) Additionally, it may provide more accurate information that reflects the needs of the older population with mental illness and their carers and families (WHO, 2008; Xavier et al., 2013).

Finally, present services for the prevention of mental illness and maintenance of general wellbeing for older adults are limited. It would be valuable for service providers to promote and prioritise prevention strategies for the most common mental illnesses suffered by older people including depression, anxiety, dementia, and substance dependence (WHO 2008). Through these prevention strategies, general pressure on the healthcare system would be reduced, allowing other areas of mental health care to more efficiently and appropriately attend to the needs of the population.

Accessibility

Due to the lack of articulation of health care, accessibility to specialised care is not facilitated by the primary care system (Caldas de Almeida et al., 2008; WHO 2008).

Additionally, Portugal still lacks community services that include specialised mental care for older adults. This is especially problematic in rural areas, in which geographical accessibility is still a challenge (Caldas de Almeida et al., 2008).

There is a need to use approaches that are specifically designed for the older population. Clinical services and research are not currently coordinated, resulting in an inadequate quality of data and training. Additionally, there is a lack of professionals with specific gerontological and geriatric expertise in mental health care (Jané-Llopis and Anderson, 2006; WHO, 2008). It may be beneficial to provide benefits which attract people to work in these areas considering that the need for geriatric specialists is growing.

The reasons for these pertinent gaps are not always clear, but they may be due to generalised national complacency by decision makers and subsequent passive acceptance by the older population regarding older age mental health services. Additionally, this complacency and acceptance may well be a sign of double discrimination of ageism and mental illness (Santana, 2000; WHO, 2008). To improve the outcomes of elderly Portuguese suffering mental illness, it would be valuable to develop specific, impartial, proactive, cohesive, and competent mental health services (WHO, 2008; Xavier et al., 2013). These services should anticipate the needs of this population, be equipped to treat, and then finally support the reintegration of older adults back into the community.

Conclusion

Portuguese society is rapidly ageing. Considering the current demographic changes and the needs of the older population, there are new challenges to face and an integrated model of mental health must be developed. Professionals in mental health care, older adults, caregivers, policy-makers and researchers should combine efforts to warrant the mental health of older people and the quality of health care. In sum, this chapter provides valuable support for increased understanding of the Portuguese mental health context and the main needs of older adults with mental disorders in Portugal, which would therefore contribute to a positive ageing experience while reducing costs to society.

References

Almeida, L. and Quintão, S. (2012). Depressão e ideação suicida em idosos institucionalizados e não institucionalizados em Portugal [Depression and suicidal ideation in elderly institutionalized and non-institutionalized in Portugal], *Acta Medica Portuguesa, 25*(6), 350-358.

Alves, S., Teixeira, L., Azevedo, M. J., Duarte, M., Paúl, C. (2015). Effectiveness of a psychoeducational programme for informal caregivers of older adults. *Scandinavian Journal Caring Science.* [Epub ahead of print] http://dx.doi.org/10.1111/scs.12222.

Anderson, D. (2007). *The Human rights of older persons in healthcare. Response from the Faculty of Old Age Psychiatry of the Royal College of Psychiatrists, Eighteenth Report.* London: Royal College of Psychiatrists.

Barak, B. (2009). Age identity: A cross-cultural global approach. *International Journal of Behavioral Development, 33,* 2–11. http://dx.doi.org/10.1177/0165025408099485.

Brayne, C., Fox, C. and Boustani, M. (2007). Dementia screening in primary care. *Journal of the American Medical Association, 298*(20), 2409-2411. http://dx.doi.org/10.1001/jama.298.20.2409.

Bryant, C., Jackson, H. and Ames, D. (2008). The prevalence of anxiety in older adults: Methodological issues and a review of the literature. *Journal of Affective Disorders, 109*(3), 233-250. http://dx.doi.org/10.1016/j.jad.2007.11.008.

Caldas de Almeida, J. M. (2009). Portuguese National Mental Health Plan (2007–2016) Executive Summary. *Mental Health in Family Medicine, 6*(4), 233–244.

Caldas de Almeida, J. M., Xavier, M. and Mateus, P. (2008). *Portugal - Country Summary. Effective and human mental health. Treatment and care for all.* Lisboa: Coordenação Nacional para a Saúde Mental.

Caltagirone, C., Perri, R., Carlesimo, G. and Fadda, L. (2001). Early detection and diagnosis of dementia. *Archives of Gerontology and Geriatrics, 33*, 67-75. http://dx.doi.org/10.1016/S0167-4943(01)00122-4.

Centro de Estudos e Desenvolvimento Regional e Urbano and Boston Consulting Group. (2008). *Study to address the needs of the senior population in Portugal - Final report.* Lisbon: Author.

Cornwell, B., Schumm, L. P., Laumann, E. O., Kim, J. and Kim, Y. J. (2014). Assessment of social network change in a national longitudinal survey. *Journals of Gerontology, Series B: Psychological Sciences and Social Sciences, 69*(8), S75-S82http://dx.doi.org/:10.1093/geronb/gbu037.

European Opinion Research Group. (2003). *The Mental Health Status of the European Population.* Brussels: DG SANCO.

European Research Infrastructure Consortium (2011). *Survey on Health, Ageing and Retirement in Europe (SHARE). Preliminary data – 2011 –first wave in Portugal.* Retrieved from http://www.share-project.org/data-access-documentation/research-data-center-data-access.html.

Frade, J., Barbosa, P. Cardoso, S. and Nunes, C. (2015). Depression in the elderly: symptoms in institutionalised and non-institutionalised individuals. *Revista de Enfermagem Referência, 4*(4), 41-48. http://dx.doi.org/10.12707/RIV14030.

Garcia, A., Passos, A., Campo, A., Pinheiro, E., Barroso, F., Coutinho, … Sholl-Franco, A. (2006). A depressão e o processo de envelhecimento [Depression and the ageing process]. *Ciências and Cognição, 7*, 111-121.

Gelder, M., Mayou, R. and Geddes, J. (2006). *Psychiatry.* Oxford: Oxford University Press.

General-Directorate for Intervention on Addictive Behaviours and Dependencies (SICAD). (2014). 2014 National Report to the EMCDDA by the Reitox National Focal Point: PORTUGAL: New Development, Trends (Lisbon, Portugal: 2014). Retrieved from http://www. emcdda.europa.eu/publications/national-reports/portugal-2014 - See more at: http://www.drugwarfacts.org/cms/Portugal#sthash. PB0swEHE.dpuf.

Goudie, F. (2002). Physical and emotional problems in later life. In G. Stokes and F. Goudie (Eds.), *The essential dementia care handbook* (pp. 22-32). Milton Keynes: Speechmark,

Gusmão, R. M., Xavier, M., Heitor, M. J., Bento, A. and Almeida, J. M. (2005). Depressive disorder burden: Global epidemiological issues and information needs in Portugal. *Acta Medica Portuguesa, 18*(2), 129-146.

Hoff, A. (2008). *Tackling poverty and social exclusion of older people – Lessons from Europe*. Oxford: Oxford Institute of Ageing.

Minghelli, B., Tomé, B, Nunes, C., Neves, A. and Simões, C. (2013). Comparison of levels of anxiety and depression among active and sedentary elderly. *Revista de Psiquiatria Clínica, 40(2),* 71-7.

Instituto Nacional de Estatística. (2011). A população estrangeira em Portugal – Destaque [The Foreigner population in Portugal -Highlight] Retrieved from file:///C:/Users/Sofia/Downloads/17PopEstPort2011%20(2).pdf.

Jané-Llopis, E. and Anderson, P. (2006). *Mental health promotion and mental disorder prevention across European Member States: a collection of country stories.* Luxembourg: European Communities.

Kovess-Masféty, V., Wiersma, D., Xavier, M., Almeida, J. M. C., Carta, M. G., Dubuis, J., ... Walsh, D. (2006). Needs for care among patients with schizophrenia in six European countries: a one-year follow-up study. *Clinical Practical Epidemiology Mental Health, 2,* 22. http://dx.doi.org/10.1186/1745-0179-2-22.

Löckenhoff, C. E., De Fruyt, F., Terracciano, A., McCrae, R. R., De Bolle, M., Costa, P. T. Jr., Aguilar-Vafaie, M. E.,... Yik, M. (2009). Perceptions of aging across 26 cultures and their culture-level associates. *Psychology Aging*, *24*(4), 941–954. http://dx.doi.org/10.1037/a0016901.

Melchiorre, M. G., Chiatti, C., Lamura, G., Torres-Gonzales, F., Stankunas, M., Lindert, J., ... Soares, J. F. J. (2013). Social support, Socio-economic status, health and abuse among older people in seven European countries. *PLOS ONE, 8*(1), e54856. http://dx.doi.org/10.1371/journal. pone.0054856.

Menninger, J. (2002). Assessment and treatment of alcoholism and substance-related disorders in the elderly. *Bulletin of the Menninger Clinic*, *66*(2), 166-83. http://dx.doi.org/10.1521/bumc.66.2.166.23364.

Minayo, M. C. S. and Cavalcante, F. G. (2010). Suicide in elderly people: a literature review. *Revista Saúde Pública, 44*(4), 750-757. http://dx.doi.org/10.1590/S0034-89102010000400020.

Minghelli, B., Tomé, B., Nunes, C., Neves, A. and Simões, C. (2013). Comparison of levels of anxiety and depression among active and sedentary elderly. *Archives of Clinical Psychiatry*, *40*(2), 71-76. http://dx.doi.org/10.1590/S0101-60832013000200004.

Nunes, B., Silva, R. D., Cruz, V. T., Roriz, J. M., Pais, J. and Silva, M. C. (2010). Prevalence and pattern of cognitive impairment in rural and urban populations from Northern Portugal. *BMC Neurology, 10*(42). http://dx.doi.org/*10,* 42. 10.1186/1471-2377-10-42.

Oliveira, K. L., Santos, A., Cruvinel, M. and Néri, A. L. (2006). Relação entre ansiedade, depressão e desesperança entre grupos de idosos [Relation between depression and lack of hope in elderly groups]. *Psicologia em Estudo, 11*, 351-359. http://dx.doi.org/10.1590/S1413-737220060 00200014.

Passos, J., Sequeira, C. and Fernandes, L. (2012). The needs of older people with mental health problems: A particular focus on dementia patients and their carers. *International Journal of Alzheimer's Disease,* 1-7. http://dx.doi.org/10.1155/2012/638267.

Paúl, C., Fonseca, A. M., Martin, I. and Amado, J. (2003). Psychosocial profile of rural and urban elders in Portugal. *European Psychologist, 8,* 160-167. http://dx.doi.org/10.1027//1016-9040.8.3.160.

Permanent Mission of Portugal to the United Nations. (2011). *Portugal's views on the situation of the rights of older persons.* Retrieved from http://www.ohchr.org/Documents/Issues/OlderPersons/Submissions/Portugal.pdf.

Piercy, K. W., Fauth, E. B., Norton, M. C., Pfister, R., Corcoran, C. D., Rabins, P. V., ... Tschanz, J. T. (2013). Predictors of dementia caregiver depressive symptoms in a population: the Cache County dementia progression study. *The Journals of Gerontology Series B: Psychological Sciences and Social Sciences, 68*(6), 921-926. http://dx.doi.org/10.1093/geronb/gbs116.

Pimentel, A. F., Afonso, R. M and Pereira, H. (2012). Depression and support in old age. *Psicologia, Saúde and Doenças, 13(2),* 311-327.

Pinqüart, M. and Sörensen, S. (2003). Differences between caregivers and noncaregivers in psychological health and physical health: a meta-analysis. *Psychology and Aging 18*(2), 250-267. http://dx.doi.org/10.1037/0882-7974.18.2.250.

Pinqüart, M. and Sörensen, S. (2005). Ethnic differences in stressors, resources, and psychological outcomes of family caregiving: A meta-analysis. *The Gerontologist, 45,* 90-106.

Ponte, C. Alemeida, V. and Fernandes, L. (2014). Suicidel ideation, depression and quality of life in the elderly: Study in a Gerentophsychiatric Consultation. *The Spanish Journal of Psychology, 17,* E14. http://dx.doi.org/10.1017/sjp. 2014.15.

Quintão, S., Costa, S., Alves, S. and Gusmão, R. (2013). Suicide after 65 years old: Current data in Portugal. In A. L. Oliveira, C. M. C. Vieira, M. P. Lima, L. Alcoforado, S. M. Ferreira and J. A. Ferreira (Eds.), *Promoting conscious and active learning and aging: How to face current and future challenges?* (pp. 321-333). Coimbra: Imprensa da Universidade de Coimbra.

Ryan, P. and Coughlan. B. J. (2013). *Ageing and older adult mental health: Issues and implications for practice.* New York, NY: Routledge.

Sampaio, D. and Telles-Correia, D. (2013). Suicídio nos Mais Velhos: Fundamental Não Esquecer! [Suicide in the Elderly: Crucial Not to Forget!] *Acta Médica Portuguesa, 26*(1), 1-2.

Santana, P. (2000). Ageing in Portugal: regional iniquities in health and health care. *Social Science and Medicine, 50,* 1025-1036. http://dx.doi.org/10.1016/S0277-9536(99)00352-4.

Santos, M. J. H. (2006). *Report on the expert workshop on "Mental Health – health Promotion and Prevention Strategies in Portugal"* organised as part of the project "Implementation of Mental health Promotion and Prevention Policies and Strategies in EU Member States and Applicant Countries (EMIP). Lisbon: Author.

Sequeira, C. (2013). Difficulties, coping strategies, satisfaction and burden in informal Portuguese caregivers. *Journal Clinical Nursing, 22*(3-4), 491-500. http://dx.doi.org/10.1111/jocn.12108.

Sociedade Portuguesa de Suicidologia. (2009). Number of suicides by age group and gender. Retrieved from http://www.spsuicidologia.pt/sobre-o-suicidio/estatistica.

Unidade de Missão dos Cuidados Continuados Integrados. (2012). *Relatório de Monitorização da actividade da RNCCI. 1º Semestre de 2012* [Report for the Monitoring of Activities of RNCCI. 1 Semester from 2012]. Lisbon: Author.

Veríssimo, M. T. (2006). *Avaliação multidimensional do Idoso.* Lisboa: Editora Psiquiatria Clínica.

von Humboldt, S., Leal, I. and Pimenta, F. (2012). Assessing subjective age and adjustment to aging in a Portuguese and German older population: A comparative multiple correspondence analysis. *International Journal of Psychological Studies, 4*(2), 141-153. http://dx.doi.org/10.5539/ijps.v4n2p141.

von Humboldt, S. and Leal, I. (2012). Building bridges: Person-centered therapy with older adults. *European Journal of Business and Social Sciences, 1*(8), 23-32.

von Humboldt, S., Leal, I. and Pimenta, F. (2014). Does spirituality really matter? – A study on the potential of spirituality to older adult's adjustment to aging. *Japanese Psychological Research, 56*, 114-125. http://dx.doi.org/10.1111/jpr.12033.

Wall, K., Aboim, S., Cunha, V. and Vasconcelos, P. (2001). Families and informal support networks in Portugal: The reproduction of inequality. *Journal of European Social Policy, 11*, 213-233.

Washburn, A. M. and von Humboldt, S. (2013). Counselling with older adults. In M. Cooper, M. O'Hara, P. F. Schmid and A. C. Bohart (Eds.), *The Handbook of person-centered psychotherapy and counseling* (2nd ed.) (pp. 297-312). New York, NY: Palgrave MacMillan.

Wetherell, J. L., Lenze, E. J. and Stanley, M. A. (2005). Evidence-based treatments of geriatric anxiety disorders. *Psychiatric Clinics of North American, 28*, 871-896. http://dx.doi.org/10.1016/j.psc.2005.09.006.

World Health Organization. (2008). *Policies and practices for mental health in Europe. Meeting the challenges.* Copenhagen, Denmark: WHO Regional Office for Europe.

World Health Organization. (2011). *World Health Statistics 2011. Geneve,* Switzerland: Author.

Wittchen, H. and Jacobi, F. (2005). Size and burden of mental disorders in Europe – a critical review and appraisal of 27 studies. *European Neuropsychopharmacology, 15*(4), 357-376.

Xavier, M., Ferraz, M., Trendi, C., et al. (2001). Transtorno de ansiedade generalizada em idosos com 80 anos ou mais [Anxiety disorder in elderdy aged 80 years old and above]. *Revista Saude Publica, 35*(3), 294-302.

Xavier, M., Baptista, H., Mendes, J. M., Magalhães, P. and Caldas de Almeida, J. M. (2013). Implementing the World Mental Health Survey Initiative in Portugal – rationale, design and fieldwork procedures. *International Journal of Mental Health Systems, 7*(19). http://dx.doi.org/10.1186/1752-4458-7-19.

Part II: High and Medium Human Development Countries

In: Ageing and Mental Health: Global Perspectives
Editors: Wendy Wen Li, Sherry M. Cummings et al.
ISBN: 978-1-63484-777-3

Chapter 10

AGED CARE AND MENTAL HEALTH IN CHINA

Wendy Wen Li[1,*], Xuewei Huang[2], Yan Chen[3] and Hongyu Li[2]
[1]James Cook University, Townsville City, QLD, Australia
[2]Guangdong Pharmaceutical University, Guangzhou, Guangdong Province, China
[3]University of Eastern Finland, Joensuu, Finland

ABSTRACT

China has the largest number of older people in the world. Strongly influenced by filial piety (respect and care for older people), Chinese elders have been historically honoured as wise and contributing members of society who deserve, and are to be provided with, care and respect. Adult children are traditionally expected to live with their ageing parents to provide financial, physical, and emotional support. As a result of the one-child policy implemented in the 1970s, the proportion of older Chinese people has increased. The traditional practice of adult children living with their ageing parents, however, has evolved, resulting in empty-nest households becoming more and more prevalent in China. Along with rapid economic development and urbanisation, the phenomenon of empty-nest has impacts on the mental health of older Chinese people who may experience loneliness, isolation, and even anxiety and depression. As there has been a lack of national investigation on the prevalence of anxiety, depression, dementia and other forms of mental disorders among older people, this chapter reviews the academic research into mental disorder prevalence. Based on the discussion of policy and available services, the chapter provides recommendations related to older adults' mental health.

Keywords: filial piety, caregiving, anxiety, depression, dementia, urbanisation

* Corresponding author: Wendy Li, James Cook University, Townsville City QLD 4811, Australia. E-mail: wendy.li@jcu.edu.au.

INTRODUCTION

China has the largest elderly population and is also one of the most rapidly ageing societies in the world (Zhao et al., 2013). According to the 2010 Census, the total population of China was 1,370,536,875 persons, of which the population of the mainland of China (excluding Hong Kong, Macau, and Taiwan) was 1,339,724,852 persons. Among these, the number of people aged 60 and over was 178 million, accounting for 13.3% of the population. The number of people aged 65 years and older was 119 million, accounting for 8.9% of the population. In 2010, % of the population was in the under-15-years age group, decreasing from 23% in 2000, while the number of people in the age group of 60 and over increased by 2.9% (National Bureau of Statistics of China, 2011). These figures suggest that life expectancy in China is increasing; however, the number of young people is plummeting due to strict birth control and the one-child policy which has been enforced since the late 1970s.

The ageing situation has posed great challenges to sustainable economic and social development in China, particularly where physical and mental health among older Chinese people is concerned. According to the National Baseline Survey of the China Health and Retirement Longitudinal Study (CHARLS; Zhao, Hu, Smith, Strauss and Yang, 2014), the first large-scale survey of those over 60 in China, physical disabilities and mental-health problems are widespread among the 17,708 respondents. Of those surveyed, 38.1% reported difficulty with daily activities and 40% showed high symptoms of depression. While 32.1% of men reported high levels of depressive symptoms, 47.6% of women reported high levels of depressive symptoms. The CHARLS also found that cognition declined rapidly with age and a large gender gap existed in cognitive ability especially among older people. The survey found that 88.7% of the respondents who required assistance with daily activities received it from family members. The substantial familial support reflects the strength of family support systems for older people.

Taking these factors into account, this chapter explores mental health issues, aged care, and related policies in China. To set the stage for the exploration, the ultural context of ageing and ageing issues caused by the one-child policy are first discussed. This is followed by a discussion on the prevalence of mental disorders among older Chinese people, the range of mental health services available, general caregiving and social support services for older Chinese people. The chapter closes with a critical review of the current polices in relation to older Chinese people with mental illness and the identification of gaps. Appropriate recommendations will be then suggested.

CULTURAL CONTEXT OF AGEING IN CHINA

Compared to other countries, ageing in China is culturally unique. For example, Chinese people traditionally rely on their family for aged care (Li, 2013). The family relationship in the Chinese culture is characterised by the relationship between parents and their children. The parent-child relationship is traditionally governed by the Confucian concept of filial piety and is a dominant feature of aged care in Chinese families. Filial piety refers to the traditions of respect, reverence, care, obedience, and fulfilling duties to one's parents and grandparents (Li, 2013). The strong influence of the value of filial piety means that Chinese elders have been historically honoured as wise and contributing members of society who deserve, and are to be provided with, care and respect (Chappell, 2005). It is expected that adult children live with their ageing parents to provide financial, physical and emotional support. Family resources are the main protection against poverty in old age, and with a larger proportion of older people, the financial and care demands on families will be severely stretched in the near future (Zhao, Smith and Strauss, 2014).

There are five aspects or practices that demonstrate filial piety towards ageing parents in Chinese familial aged care (Li, 2013). These are co-residence with ageing parents, support to parents, respecting parents, ancestral worship, and children's achievements. Traditionally, co-residence with one's parents was paramount in practicing filial piety and is a key indicator of filial piety. Members of a family are expected to reside under the same roof where they have obligations to share resources and to honour, venerate, and look after aged relatives. Living separately from the parental household is socially disapproved of and considered unfilial. Another key component of filial piety is physical support to one's parents. Physical support to parents includes physically looking after parents and providing material support to parents. This was of essential importance in traditional, agricultural Chinese society because few organisations existed outside the family to serve an individual's needs. Although physical and material support is regarded important for a filial child, material goods alone do not suffice. Material support without reverence does not fulfil the dictates of traditional filial piety. Paying respect to ancestors is incorporated within the belief of filial piety and manifested in mourning and ancestral worship rituals. A traditional funeral for the dead parent is regarded as a demonstration of love and respect and a way of teaching filial piety to the younger generation. High achieving children are also seen as more filial, which reflects the Confucian belief that one's duty is to make the family name known and respected thus bringing honour to the family.

While filial piety remains an important value for Chinese people, the practices of filial piety, in particular the living arrangements of older people, have evolved in the context of urbanisation, migration, and social policy in contemporary China (Li, Hodgetts, Ho and Stolte, 2010). In the past three decades, for example, China has experienced the largest urbanisation and migration in its history, leading to a significant rise in urban population from 191 million in 1980 to 622 million in 2009 (Chan, 2010). As a result of urbanisation and migration, the predominant family form in contemporary China has become nuclear. Older people reside either with a spouse only, or with a spouse and one or more unmarried children who are dependent on them (Li, 2013). Empty-nest households occupied solely by older couples are also a growing phenomenon (All-China Women's Federation, 2009). In 2003, the empty-nest family structure in China accounted for almost 25% of elderly households, and the proportion of empty-nest families in Beijing was over 35% (Li, Chen and Li, 2003). It is estimated that the proportion of empty-nest households will reach 90% of elderly households by 2030 (Xie, Zhang, Peng and Jiao, 2010). It is thus no longer obligatory for married adult children to live with their aged parents. Moreover, housing reform policies, such as privatisation of public houses in the late 1980s and the Monetarisation of Housing Reform Policy that provided subsidies to assist young people to buy their own houses, have contributed to a substantial reduction in intergenerational co-residence in China (Li, 2013).

Such changes in older people's living arrangements may make it more difficult for older Chinese adults to seek social support from their family members. Consequently, these older people are more likely to experience loneliness and disconnectedness, which may prevent them from remaining engaged in meaningful relationships. A recent study in China indicated that about 28% of older Chinese adults reported feeling lonely (Luo and Waite, 2014). Social indicators such as increased level of urbanisation, personal medical expenditure, divorce rate, and rate of unemployment were predictors of increased loneliness. Research has suggested that loneliness may increase the likelihood of mental health problems such as depressive symptoms, stress, anxiety, and anger (Chen, Conwell and Chiu, 2014). These psychological problems may in turn influence physiological functioning, such as chronic pain. The Global Burden of Disease Study showed that 33% of Chinese people aged 60 years and older had chronic pain comprising 39% of women and 28% of men. The study also found that depression was a serious problem among older Chinese people, causing not only disability but also premature death (Zhao, Hu, Smith, Strauss and Yang, 2012).

As noted previously, the increased proportion of ageing population is partly a result of China's one-child policy. The one-child policy has also contributed to the increased burden in aged care. At a micro familial level, although the filial piety practices have changed over time, a majority of older people are still cared for by their adult children. However, many nuclear families in China have morphed into the 4-2-1 (four grandparents, two parents and one child) structure (Du, 2000). When the youngest individual from a 4-2-1 family reaches working age, he/she would have to care for two ageing parents and four aged grandparents (Zhao and Gao, 2014). Such a family structure makes it difficult for the one-child couple to provide support to their aged parents and grandparents.

At a macro level, the population situation in China has undergone great changes. First, the decline in the fertility rate is much faster than expected. According to the 2010 Census the total fertility rate of women of child-bearing age is 1.18, with 0.88 for urban areas and 1.44 for rural areas. These rates are below the replacement level (Zhao and Chen, 2011), which suggests that each woman did not produce enough children to replace herself and her partner. As urbanisation continues to increase, more people living in rural areas will move to cities. In that regard, low birth rate may not only be consolidated but also further continued as the implementation of the one-child policy is stricter in cities. Secondly, the sex ratio at birth has also been distorted (Ding and Hesketh, 2006). There are 20% fewer new-born girls than new-born boys. With such a low fertility rate, the number of women of child-bearing age in the future will also decrease significantly (Zhao and Gao, 2014).

Recognising the impact of the one-child policy on the aged care system, the Chinese Government in 2013 announced a significant adjustment to the one-child policy, allowing couples to have two children if one spouse is an only child (Zhao and Gao, 2014). Although the impact of this policy on aged care remains unclear, it will definitely influence aged care in China in the near future.

Without sufficient aged-care coverage by the social welfare system, the social and economic status of older people has a significant impact on their mental health. Older people of low social and economic status may feel hopeless and helpless when they consider their future medical care. As noted previously, the rapid economic development in China brings about the phenomenon of young people seeking jobs outside the area in which their ageing parents live. These adult children may not be able to provide day-to-day care for their aged parents, let alone live with them. The gap between the expectation of the ageing parents who may expect to live with their adult children and the reality may influence the ageing parents' moods and even mental health.

Prevalence of Mental Disorders among Older Chinese Adults

As noted, China's remarkable economic growth and urbanisation together with the implementation of the one-child policy has resulted in dramatic changes in familial aged care, potentially rendering older people more financially and socially vulnerable. These changes have also increased gender and urban-rural inequality among older people. The priorities in health care and pension systems have been given to urban areas while rural communities are neglected and the prevalence of mental disorders among older people is higher than that in urban areas (Nie, Wang, Sun and Yang, 2013; Sun, Qu, Jiang, Yuan, Min and Qin, 2011; Wang, Liao, Yang, Wang and Deng, 2014). This suggests that rapid economic development has not been accompanied by improving health indicators (Woo, 2013).

Depression and Anxiety

There is a lack of national surveys on geriatric mental health in China. There are a number of academic studies that provide some understandings of prevalence of depression and anxiety among older Chinese people. A systematic review and meta-analysis on depression among community-dwelling older people living in 18 provinces in China found that 22.4% of participants reported that they had experienced depressive symptoms and the prevalence of depressive disorders was 17.2% (Nie at al., 2013). In their meta-analysis on anxiety disorders of older people in China, Su et al. (2011) found that the prevalence of anxiety disorders among people aged 55 years and over was 6.8% and 22.1% of participants reported experiencing anxiety symptoms.

A number of regional studies have also focused on investigating mental disorder rates in community samples. According to these studies, the prevalence of depression was between 3.6% and 4.33% in regional communities. The prevalence among females (5.53%) was statistically significantly higher than males (2.95%) and this prevalence increased with age. Furthermore, participants with lower education levels, lower income and poor housing conditions, childless, living in urban areas and alone, and having relationship problems with family members reflected higher rates of mental health problems than their counterparts (Sun et al., 2011; Wang et al., 2014). In relation to anxiety, Qu et al. (2010) reported that the prevalence of anxiety disorders among older people was 2.57 per cent with 2.51 per cent for males and 2.59 per cent for females. The prevalence was also higher (1.54%) in urban than rural (0.72%) areas. They found that anxiety was associated with poor housing conditions, physical illness, financial difficulties and psychological stress. The recovery rate of those with anxiety disorders was low, with as few as 9.41% experiencing a complete recovery.

Dementia

Dementia is the most common worldwide neurodegenerative disease of ageing, and 20% of patients with dementia live in China. According to previous epidemiologic investigations, the prevalence of dementia in China was thought to be between 3% and 7.5% of the elderly population, with Alzheimer's disease the majority, at a prevalence of around 2 to 4% (Chen, Hu, Wei and Wilson, 2014; Liu, Wang and Tan, 2013). Chen et al. (2014) reported that over 90% of dementia cases in China go undetected, suggesting that these figures may be hugely underestimating the actual prevalence. The prevalence of dementia in urban areas (3%) appears to be higher than in rural areas (2%) (Llibre Rodriguez et al., 2008), with a high level of undiagnosed dementia in rural areas (Chen et al., 2014). Using DSM-IV dementia diagnosis, Llibre Rodriguez et al. (2008) found that in China there was a higher prevalence of dementia among older females living in urban areas (4.3%) than their male counterpart (3.1%). An opposite trend of prevalence was observed in rural areas, with 3.4% of older males and 2.8% of older females living in rural areas diagnosed with dementia. It has been reported that dementia in China is related to socio-economic status. Older Chinese people with higher education were less likely to have dementia compared with those who were illiterate (Liu et al., 2013). It has been also observed that dementia and late-life depression were significantly associated with increased mortality (Chen et al., 2014).

Suicide

Suicide is a major issue for older Chinese people which is only gradually being recognised. Suicide in mainland China shows unique demographic patterns with age: the group aged over 65 years has the highest rate of completed suicide. Suicide prevalence among older people in China varies from a range of 0.04%to 0.2%. In comparison, the suicide rate in the general Chinese population is 0.02% while the global average is 0.01% (Li, Xiao and Xiao, 2009).

The number of rural elderly suicides largely accounts for the high national suicide rate of older people. The rural suicide prevalence among older adults is three to five times higher than the urban prevalence. Nevertheless, the female-to-male ratio of suicide between urban and rural older persons is reversed in the population aged younger than 60 years. For people aged 60 years and over, the female-to-male ratio is 1/1.1 in urban areas and 1/1.5 in rural areas. In comparison, for the younger population, female suicide rates exceed male rates by an average of 26%, with young rural female suicide rates being 66% higher than suicide rates among young rural males (Philips, Li and Zhang, 2002).

Furthermore, suicide methods and causes are different from those in Western countries. It has been found that pesticides are frequently used as substances for suicide, in particular in rural areas (Li et al., 2009). In Philips et al.'s (2002) study, of the 519 suicide cases, 323 (62%) died by ingestion of agricultural chemicals or rat poison (in 211 cases the poison was stored in the home), 104 (20%) by hanging, 35 (7%) by poisoning with other substances, 26 (5%) by drowning, 12 (2%) by jumping off a high building, and 19 (4%) by other methods.

Mental Health Services for Older People

Cultural beliefs often influence the diagnosis and treatment of mental disorders, and shape attitudes towards mental illness. The Chinese culture values conformity to norms, emotional self-control, and family recognition through achievement (Li, 2013). People with mental disorders are often stigmatised and seen as a source of shame, not only for the individual, but also for the family. As a result, mental health services in China are often under-utilised. In a study investigating mental health service demand and utilisation among 914 older people in a rural community, Ma et al. (2013) found that the prevalence of mental disorders was as high as 15.97%. However, only six out of 914 participants (two persons with mental disorders) had sought professional help to cope with their mental problems. Among the participants, 20.9% reported that they would like to know more about mental health services and 6.1% reported that they needed mental health services. These findings suggest that older Chinese people lack knowledge about mental health services. A public health approach to promoting mental health services may address this issue that older people face.

There are four main departments providing psychiatric services in China. The largest mental health care system is administered by the Ministry of Health and its local offices. This system consists of public psychiatric hospitals which provide services for citizens who have health insurance to cover the incurred treatment costs. The second largest system serves people who have no job, no home or no money to pay for health care services. This system is operated by the local bureau of the Ministry of Civil Affairs. The third mental health care system is run by the military. Although the primary targets of these services are military personnel and their families, in recent years, fee-charging services have started to be offered to civilians. Lastly, under the Ministry of Public Security, most of the provinces in China have established hospitals for admitting criminal offenders with mental health problems (Wong, Zhang, Pan and He, 2014).

Psychiatric services in China principally cover all age groups, including children, adolescents, adults and older people. As a result, mental health services for older people in China are mainly provided by hospitals that offer services to the general population. Generally speaking, there are three types of such services. Firstly, services provided by hospitals, including public and private psychiatric hospitals, general hospitals, community hospitals and welfare mental hospitals. The benefit of many psychiatric hospitals to the elderly is that they provide wards specifically for older individuals. Community hospitals are also developing and growing in China, becoming an important player in the provision of mental health services. They provide services to people who have mild psychological problems and referrals to mental health specialists. Welfare mental hospitals provide outpatient and inpatient mental health services to people who have no family members to care for them.

Secondly, there are services provided by nursing homes. Nursing homes offer services to older people who lose the ability to take care of themselves, many of which suffer from dementia. These nursing homes mainly provide daily care for older people but lack specific services for people with mental disorders, including dementia.

The emergence of private health management companies are also changing the face of aged care in China. These privately managed health facilities provide a diverse range of mental health services to the public, including mental health services specifically for older people. These include psychological counselling and psychotherapy. If these private services develop steadily and pay more attention to geriatric mental health services, they may make a significant contribution to mental health services for older people. However, for these private mental health services, out-of-pocket costs remain high due to high costs and limited insurance coverage in private health services.

In recent decades, China has launched a series of policy initiatives to improve its health care and social security systems. In order to improve the equity of health service utilisation for urban residents, the Chinese government established two basic medical insurance schemes for urban residents: the Urban Employee Basic Medical Insurance scheme (UEBMI) implemented in 1999 and the Urban Resident Basic Medical Insurance scheme (URBMI) implemented in 2007. The UEBMI covers employees and retirees from enterprises and public institutions, whilst the other urban residents, including the unemployed, children and students, are covered by the URBMI. By the end of 2012, more than 37% and 33% of people were covered by UEBMI and URBMI respectively across the country (Zhou et al., 2014). In 2003, China adopted the New Cooperative Medical Scheme (NCMS) in rural areas where 80% of people were without health insurance of any kind. Beginning with only 310 out of China's 2861 rural counties in 2004, its coverage had expanded to 2451 counties by the end of 2007, accounting for 86% of all rural counties in China (Lei and Lin, 2009). In 2009, the New Rural Pension Insurance pilot programme covered 10% of Chinese counties and is scheduled to roll out nationwide to cover all rural elderly by 2020 (Feng et al., 2012). However, these schemes have limited coverage especially for patients who seek private mental health services. The out-of-pocket costs of private mental health care are therefore still very expensive for many families even if they have health insurance.

FAMILIAL, COMMUNITY AND INSTITUTIONAL CAREGIVING FOR OLDER PEOPLE

Family caregiving is the main caregiving category in contemporary China (Wu, 2010). It is a general expectation of Chinese parents that they will be looked after by their adult children in their old age (Chen, 2000). This is reflected in the Chinese saying: 'raising children to provide for old age.'

To strengthen familial caregiving, looking after ageing parents is prescribed by the *Law on Protection of the Rights and Interests of the Aging China* (The Standing Committee of the National People's Congress, 2013). The Law states that aged care is established upon the belief that family members should respect, concern and care for the elders in the family.

Familial caregiving has its advantages. For example, older people can be taken care of by family members who understand the ageing family members' habits, routines and demands much better than caregivers external to the family. Moreover, emotional support from family members could be an effective way to prevent older people from developing mental disorders and promote their physical and mental well-being in turn (Chen, 2000). Intergenerational reciprocal support can also be achieved through family caregiving. For example, adult children offer emotional support to their parents while their parents provide help with childcare and with other household chores (Li, 2013).

Due to the unbalanced and different social security systems between rural and urban areas, the proportion of people who receive family caregiving is much higher in rural than in urban areas (Li, 2006). The social benefits in rural areas are extremely low compared to those in urban areas. For instance, in 2007, the average standard of minimum 'urban living guarantee' was 182.4 RMB (approximately 24USD) per person a month in urban areas and only 70 RMB (approximately 9USD) per person in rural areas (Xu, 2011). Older people in rural areas do not have sufficient savings to financially support their daily living costs in their old age. They thus have to rely on their children for financial support and caregiving.

Another unique feature of older people in China as compared to their counterparts in Western countries is the phenomenon of them ageing before getting rich. In westerns countries, population ageing happened only after having a highly developed economy which has entered a stable period. In other words, ageing after getting rich is the feature of population ageing in Western countries. On the contrary, the process of population ageing and economic development occurs simultaneously in China (Zhao and Gao, 2014). The phenomenon of 'ageing before getting rich,' therefore, has enormous financial burden on family members who are primary caregivers to their aged family members. Family caregiving to some extent transfers the burden of the social support system to the families, reducing the aged care pressure on the Chinese Government, which is particularly beneficial considering that the governmental ageing support system is under developed (Xia, 2012; Chen, 2000).

To better support older people, community caregiving is growing in China. Community caregiving provides services that support older people in staying home in their later lives, offering low-level care within a person's home for those who require basic support and assistance with daily activities. The services include household cleaning, shelter service, psychological counselling, cultural entertainment activities, elderly marriage service and palliative care (Mu, 2000). Community caregiving is welcomed by older people because it provides services which support older people in remaining in a familiar living environment while receiving social service. However, community caregiving in China lacks support for older people with mental health disorders. There is also a lack of policies and funding that support the community to provide services to older people with mental health problems.

Apart from familial and community support, institutional care is another emerging form of caregiving in urban China, which includes nursing homes and charity houses. Such institutions provide daily care, medical care and emotional support to their residents. Past decades have seen institutional caregiving becoming more popular among older people living in urban areas. However, many older people are reluctant to move to institutional care. For instance, Deng et al. (2003) reported that, in their study on older people's caregiving modes, 54.9% of older people were not willing to go to institutions. According to Li and Gong (2014), institutional aged care facilities for people aged 65 and over are significantly insufficient. For example, as of 2010 there were an estimated 40,000 elder care facilities and 3.15 million beds in those facilities nationwide. On a per capita basis, China has about half as many long-term care beds per 1,000 older people as most developed countries do. However, only 1.5-2.0% of people aged 65 and over live in residential care facilities in China, compared with 4-8% in Western countries (Feng, Liu, Guan and Mor, 2012). The following factors may contribute to this phenomenon. Firstly, sending aged parents to institutional care may be regarded as unfilial behaviour. Many older Chinese people expect to be looked after by their own children rather than by staff members in an institutional care facility when they become old. They may also feel that they are being abandoned if they move to an aged care institution. Secondly, moving to a new living environment in later age is a great challenge to many older people. Older people usually have developed a sense of physical intimacy and comfort in their own house. Their own residence has been transformed into a social space through their familiarity and connections with their neighbourhood and neighbours. When they move to an aged care facility, they may experience alienation and isolation due to a lack of attachments and bonds to the new environment (Han and Li, 2013).

LAWS AND POLICIES RELATED TO OLDER PEOPLE'S MENTAL HEALTH

In 2012, the Chinese government enacted a law aimed at compelling adult children to visit their ageing parents. The law, *Protection of the Rights and Interests of Elderly People,* has nine clauses that lay out the duties of children and their obligation to attend to the spiritual needs of older people. This law also specifies that the nation state and society should take actions towards providing general and medical care for older people, and to create an environment where older people have meaningful and interesting things to learn and have enjoyment and joy (The Standing Committee of the National People's Congress, 2013). Having enjoyment and joy refers to ample cultural and physical activities that are suitable for older people's characteristics carried out by the state, governments, and society at all levels. These activities should enable people to enjoy their old age pleasantly (The Standing Committee of the National People's Congress, 2012).

The Law prescribes that children are obligated to provide mental care for their parents, and this is a remarkable change. It states that family members have to be concerned about the older people's mental requirement and cannot place their older family members in a neglected and isolated situation; adult children living separately from their ageing parents need to visit or greet their parents frequently. Failing to visit parents frequently is regarded as illegal conduct. To support this, the Law also requires that organisations should guarantee carers' rights by allowing employees to take leave and visit parents. It is heartening to see that the Law makes filial duty a legal matter as it attempts to address the spiritual needs of older people, which is a gap in China's social welfare system that mainly focuses on the material needs of the elders. However, the Law does not stipulate any punishments for people who neglect their parents. The impact of the Law remains unclear due to the short period of enforcement and warrants future research.

China's first national mental health legislation, the *Mental Health Law of the People's Republic of China*, was adopted by the Standing Committee of the National People's Congress in 2012, with the law taking effect in 2013 (The Standing Committee of the National People's Congress, 2012). Although this Mental Health Law is not specifically targeted at older people, it is applicable for older people who suffer from mental illness. The Law fundamentally transforms the provision of mental health services in China by requiring psychiatric treatment to be voluntary in the majority of circumstances. Traditionally, families in China are responsible for the care of disabled family members. The decision of whether an individual is treated for a mental disorder, particularly if it involves inpatient treatment, is usually made by family members, instead of by the individual who suffers a mental disorder or by the treating psychiatrist. As more treatment services have become available for less severe forms of mental disorders in China, there has been an increase in the number of individuals voluntarily seeking outpatient services without the involvement of their families. Nevertheless, the majority of individuals with severe mental disorders who require inpatient treatment are still involuntarily admitted by their legal guardians who are usually family members. Changing such long-standing practice to a largely voluntary admission system in the Law will increase the burden on families. This is because family members are legally responsible for the care and management of patients who refuse voluntary inpatient treatment and bear civil liability for the patients' behaviour which may indulge in self-harm or in harming others. The conversion of an involuntary to a voluntary admission system in hospitals will also greatly increase the need for community-based mental health services. As noted previously, these services are currently weak in most urban communities and absent in most rural communities (Phillips et al., 2013).

POLICY AND SERVICE GAPS IN CHINA'S MENTAL HEALTH SYSTEM FOR OLDER PEOPLE AND RECOMMENDATIONS

As discussed previously, the current delivery system and service provision of mental health care for older people in China is insufficient for the needs of mental health aged care. Currently, the Chinese mental health-care system is dominated by large psychiatric hospitals that provide inpatient treatment for severe mental illness. There is a lack of preventive or community-based mental health services. There is also a lack of networks for psychological rehabilitation for the mental health patients and their families (Li, Sunb, Zhang, Shi and Kolstad, 2014).

As pointed out by Philips et al. (2013), the *Mental Health Law of the People's Republic of China* reflects a significant turning point for psychiatry in China, and potentially for global mental health. At present, the central government has both the political will and the resources available to implement the changes required by the Law. What is uncertain is whether or not the political will and resources will be sustained in the long term. More importantly, it remains unclear whether local agencies, particularly those in less affluent rural areas, have the motivation and resources needed to implement the required changes. It is also uncertain whether the monitoring system put in place will be sufficiently comprehensive and of sufficient quality to accurately assess the effect of the Law over time. A comprehensive and high quality monitoring system is essentially important as it provides the information needed to make necessary midcourse corrections.

Furthermore, as in the West, educational programmes in the areas of ageing and care of older people with mental disorders are needed for physicians, nurses, and other healthcare professionals. These programmes should focus on principles and practices related to geriatric mental health, not just about age-related diseases common in older people. The programmes will ensure that people working with older adults with mental health disorders have the minimum qualifications. Education programmes aiming to improve mental health literacy among older people are also needed. Currently, there is lack of empirical knowledge about the mental health literacy of older people in China, and this lack of information is hindering the development of health promotion programmes. As a result, poor 'mental health literacy,' namely, poor knowledge and understanding of the nature and treatment of mental health problems, is a major factor in low or inappropriate treatment-seeking among individuals with mental health problems (Jorm, 2000, 2012), and greatly contributes to the low level of utilisation of mental health services. Efforts are therefore needed to identify specific aspects of mental health literacy in different demographic subgroups of older Chinese people and to use that knowledge to develop health promotion programmes for this population.

CONCLUSION

Population ageing in China has many unique features. In addition to the cultural aged-care values of filial piety, these factors significantly influence mental health caregiving of older people. As China has the largest number of older people in the world and a large number of older people suffering from mental health disorders such as depression, anxiety, and dementia, more investment is needed to offer preventive, community-based mental health, and long-term aged care services. Furthermore, government policy needs to incorporate deeper, long-term benefits as opposed to the shallow, short term benefits seen in present policy. Gender and urban-rural health inequalities in aged care also need to be addressed in order to improve mental health overall. Further development of educational programmes in the areas of ageing, mental health literacy and care of older people with mental disorders is urgently needed.

REFERENCES

All-China Women's Federation. (2009). *Filial piety in contemporary China*. Retrieved from http://www.womenofchina.cn/Data_Research/Latest_Statistics/211564.jsp.

Chan, K. W. (2010). China's city population statistics and implications for economic analysis [in Chinese]. In: C. Fang (Ed.), *Reports on China's population and labor No. 11: Labor market challenges in the post-crisis era* (pp. 236-247). Beijing, China: Social Science Academic Press.

Chappell, N. L. (2005). Perceived change in quality of life among Chinese Canadian seniors: The role of involvement in Chinese culture. *Journal of Happiness Studies*, 6, 69-91.

Chen, S. (2000). Research review on Chinese caregiving forms for older people [in Chinese]. *Population Journal*, 3(1), 34-36.

Chen, S., Conwell, Y., and Chiu, H. (2014). Loneliness and aging in China - A public health problem in need of solutions. *International Psychogeriatrics,* 26(11), 1771–1772.

Chen, R., Hu, Z., Wei, L, and Wilson, K. (2014). Socioeconomic status and survival among older adults with dementia and depression. *The British Journal of Psychiatry*, 204, 436-440.

Deng, Y., Li, N. X, Liu, C. J., Wang Y., Wu, X. P., and Yang, W. Z. (2003). Study of influencial factors on older people's selecting caregiving modes [in Chinese]. *Chinese Journal of Public Health*, 19(6), 731-732.

Ding, Q., and Hesketh, T. (2006). Family size, fertility preference and sex ratio in China in the era of the one child family policy: Results from National Family Planning and Reproductive Health Survey. *British Medical Journal*, 333, 371-373.

Du, P. (2000). *Atlas of Ageing Population in Beijing* [in Chinese]. Beijing, China: China Population Publishing House.

Feng, Z., Liu, C., Guan, X., and Mor, V. (2012). China's rapidly aging population creates policy challenges in shaping a viable long-term care system. *Global Health*, 12, 2764-2773.

Han, B. X., and Li, J. (2013). Scientific study on mental health research and promotion of aged population [in Chinese]. *Scientific Research on Aging*, 1(4), 8-17.

Jorm, A. F. (2000). Mental health literacy: Public knowledge and beliefs about mental health disorders. *The British Journal of Psychiatry*, 177, 396-401.

Jorm, A. F. (2012). Mental health literacy: Empowering the community to take action for better mental health. *American Psychologist*, 67(3), 231-243.

Lei, X., and Ling, W. (2009). The new cooperative medical scheme in rural China: Does more coverage mean more service and better health. *Health Economics*, 18, S25-S46.

Llibre Rodriguez, J., Ferri, C., Acosta, D., Guerra, M., Huang, Y., Jacob, K. ... Prince, M. (2008). Prevalence of dementia in Latin America, India, and China: a population-based cross-sectional survey. *Lancet*, 372, 464-474.

Li, D. M., Chen, T. Y., and Li, G. Y. (2003). The problem of mental health in the elderly in empty-nest family [in Chinese]. *Chinese Journal of Gerontology*, 23, 405-407.

Li, K., Sun, X., Zhang, Y., Shi, G., and Kolstad, A. (2014). Mental health care in China: review on the delivery and policy issues in 1949-2009 and the outlook for the next decade. *Acta Neuropsychiatrica*, 40, 134-145.

Li, W. W. (2013). *Shifting selves in migration: Home, ageing in place and wellbeing*. Beijing, China: Central Compilation and Translation Press.

Li, W. W., Hodgetts, D., Ho, E., and Stolte, O. (2010). From early Confucian texts to ageing care in China and abroad today: The evolution of filial piety and its implications. *Journal of US-China Public Administration*, 7(7), 48-59.

Li, X. Y., Xiao, Z., and Xiao, S. (2009). Suicide among the elderly in mainland China. *Psychogeriatrics*, 9, 62-66.

Li, X. Y., and Gong, C. (2014). Exploration of community model for the elderly spiritual support in urban areas [in Chinese]. *Reform and Opening*, 5, 61-62.

Li, X. Y. (2006). Analysis on the transition of rural old-age caregiving from family caregiving to social endowment [in Chinese]. *Foreign Economic Relations and Trade*, 1, 90-92.

Liu, J., Wang, L-N., and Tan, J-P. (2013). Dementia in China: current status. *Neurology*, 81, 1077-1078.

Luo, Y., and Waite, L. J. (2014). Loneliness and mortality among older adults in China. *The Journals of Gerontology, Series B: Psychological Sciences and Social Sciences*, 69, 633-645.

Ma, Y., Hu, Z., Zhu, A. R., Chen R.L., and Qin, X. (2013). Mental health service demand and utilization among older people in rural community [in Chinese]. *Chinese Rural Health Service Administration*. 33(5), 488-489.

Mu, G. Z. (2000). Reform and prospect of traditional pension plan for the aged in China [in Chinese]. *Journal of Renmin University of China*, 5, 39-44.

National Bureau of Statistics of China. (2011). *Communiqué of the National Bureau of Statistics of People's Republic of China on Major Figures of the 2010 Population Census (No. 1)*. Retrieved from http://web.archive.org/web/20131108022004/http://www.stats.gov.cn/english/newsandcomingevents/t20110428_402722244.htm.

Wong, D., Zhuang, X., Pan, J-Y, and He, X. (2014). A critical review of mental health and mental health-related policies in China: More actions required. *International Journal of Social Welfare*, 23, 195-204.

Nie, X. L., Wang, H. Y., Sun, F., and Yang Z. R. (2013). Detection rate of depression among community-dwelling older adults in China: a systematic review and updated meta-analysis of studies in 2000-2012. *Chinese Mental Health Journal*, 27(11), 805-814.

Phillips, M., Chen, H., Diesfeld, K., Xie, B., Cheng, H., Mellsop, G., and Liu, X. (2013). China's new mental health law: Reframing involuntary treatment. *American Journal of Psychiatry*. 176, 588-591.

Philips, M., Li, X., and Zhang, Y. (2002). Suicide rates in China, 1995-99. *Lancet*, 359, 835-840.

Phillips, M., Yang, G., Zhang, Y., Wang, L., Ji, H., and Zhou, M. (2002). Risk factors for suicide in China: A national case-control psychological autopsy study. *Lancet*, 360, 1728-1736.

Qu, Z. F., Yang, Z. D., Jiang, Q., Yuan, J., Qin, J., Tang, Q., … Wang, H. J. (2011). Epidemiological characteristics of anxiety disorders in elderly in Pudong New District, Shanghai: A community-based study [in Chinese]. *Chinese Journal of Clinicians*. 5(5), 223-227.

The Standing Committee of the National People's Congress. (2012). *Mental Health Law of the People's Republic of China* [in Chinese]. Retrieved from http://www.gov.cn/jrzg/2012-10/26/content_2252122.htm.

The Standing Committee of the National People's Congress. (2013). Law of the People's Republic of China on Protection of the Rights and Interests of the Elderly [in Chinese]. Retrieved from http://www.hrichina.org/en/law/law-peoples-republic-china-protection-rights-and-interests-elderly.

Sun, X. R., Qu, Z. F., Jiang, Q., Yuan, J., Min, J., and Qin, H.Y. (2011). Investigation of the Epidemiology of Senile Depression in Community of Pudong New Area, Shanghai [in Chinese]. *Medical Journal of Chinese People's Health*, 23(9), 1078-1119.

Wang W. W., Liao X. Y., Yang, Z. Y., Wang, X., and Deng, W. Q. (2014). Depression of elderly residents in the central districts of Chengdu City: A study on epidemiological screening and risk factors. *Chines Journal of Evidence-based Medicine*, 14(1), 21-24.

Wong, D., Zhuang, X., Pan, J-Y, and He, X. (2014). A critical review of mental health and mental health-related policies in China: More actions required. *International Journal of Social Welfare*, 23, 195-204.

Woo, J. (2013). Meeting the needs of an aging population in China: Public health and policy implications. *Journal of Clinical Gerontology and Geriatrics*, 4, 31-32.

Wu, C. P. (2010). Urban Women's Pension and Strategic Choice [in Chinese]. *Journal of Anhui Normal University (Humilities. and Social Sciences)*, 1, 40-44.

Xia, L. (2012). *Study on selection of diversified ageing caregiving modes* [in Chinese]. Unpublished master's thesis, Zhejiang University of Finance and Economics, Hangzhou, China.

Xie, B. (2012). Where is the path to recovery when psychiatric hospitalization becomes too difficult? *Shanghai Archives of Psychiatry*, 24, 38-40.

Xie, L. Q., Zhang, J. P., Peng, F., and Jiao, N. N. (2010). Prevalence and related influencing factors of depressive symptoms for empty-nest elderly living in the rural area of YongZhou, China. *Archives of Gerontology and Geriatrics*, 50(1), 24-29.

Xu, Y. (2010). Research of China's urban and rural social security system under the perspective of equity [in Chinese]. *Review on Applied Economics*, 1, 161-163.

Zhao, Z. W. And Chen, W. (2011). China's far below-replacement fertility and its long-term impact: Comments on the preliminary results of the 2010 Census. *Demographic Research*, 25, 817-836.

Zhao, S., and Gao, Y. (2014). Can adjustments of China's family planning policy truly relieve pressures arising from population aging? *International Journal of China Studies*, 5(3), 657-680.

Zhao, Y., Hu, Y., Smith, J. P., Strauss, J., and Yang, G. (2014). Cohort profile: the China Health and Retirement Longitudinal Study (CHARLS). *International Journal of Epidemiology*, 43, 61-68.

Zhao, Y., Park, A., Strauss, J., Giles, J., Mao, S., Crimmins, E., … Yin, X. (2013). *Challenges of population aging in China: Evidence from the national baseline survey of the China health and retirement longitudinal study (CHARLS).* Beijing, China: The CHARLS Research.

Zhao, Y., Smith, J. P., and Strauss, J. (2014). Can china age healthily? *Lancet*. 384, 723-724.

Zhou Z., Liang, L., Zhou, Z., Li, Z., Gao, J., and Chen, G. (2014). The effects of China's urban basic medical insurance schemes on the equity of health service utilization: evidence from Shaanxi Province. *International Journal for Equity in Health*, 13, 23-33.

In: Ageing and Mental Health: Global Perspectives
Editors: Wendy Wen Li, Sherry M. Cummings et al.
ISBN: 978-1-63484-777-3

Chapter 11

GERONTOLOGICAL MENTAL HEALTH IN INDIA

***Ilango Ponnuswami*[1,*] *and P. Udhayakumar*[2]**
[1]Bharathidasan University, Tiruchirappalli, Tamil Nadu, India
[2]Central University of Tamil Nadu, Thiruvarur, Tamil Nadu, India

ABSTRACT

India is witnessing a steady increase in old age population. The robust growth in the number of elderly people in the general population in recent years is termed the "graying of the world." As the older population is more vulnerable to mental health related problems, the number of older persons with mental health problems is expected to increase in the near future. Organizing geriatric mental health services for the Indian old age population is indeed a daunting task. Lack of awareness, inadequate training opportunities, scarcity of mental health personnel, 'brain drain', and the stigma of seeking help for problems related to mental health are some of the challenges of geriatric psychiatry in the future in India. This chapter looks at the gerontological mental health scenario in India with regard to mental health care policies and services. It discusses old age psychiatry in India, the epidemiology of mental health problems, mental health service needs, delivery of appropriate services within the mental health policy framework, integration of geriatric mental health care into the already existing mental health care service delivery system and training for professionals already working or wishing to work in the field of gerontological mental health.

Keywords: gerontology, geriatric mental health, old age psychiatry, mental health, older persons

* Corresponding author: Email: pon.ilango@gmail.com.

INTRODUCTION

"Aging is not lost youth but a new stage of opportunity and strength"

Betty Friedan

These words describe the feeling of most of the elderly in India. Ever since independence, the country has been passing through a phase of rapid transition in almost all areas, be it social, demographic, health care, or economic. The transformed India is faced with newer challenges in almost all walks of life. A very rapidly emerging issue relates to developing services and care for the grey segment of the population whose numbers are growing every year (Tiwari and Pandey, 2012). India's population is growing older. As of 2011, with an estimated population of 1.21 billion, India is the world's second most populated country after China (Chandramouli, 2011). It accounted for more than 17% of the world's population in 2011 according to the estimates prepared by the United Nations (United Nations, 2011). It was estimated that by 2050, the overall population in India will grow by 55% and the population aged 60 years and above will increase by 26% (United Nations, 2002). This has resulted in an increased proportion of older people in the total population, termed, the "greying of population" (Prakash and Kukreti, 2013). Rapid growth in the percentage and proportion of older adults in the country is associated with major consequences and implications in all areas of day-to-day life (Tiwari and Pandey, 2012). The old age population is more vulnerable to health related problems including mental illness. Various prevalence studies have reported mental health problems among older adults to be much higher compared to other age groups (Ramachandran et al., 1979; Reddy and Chandrashekhar, 1998; Tiwari, 2000; Tiwari et al., 2010). Older people are regarded as one of the vulnerable populations in the field of health. Vulnerable populations are defined as being at risk of poor physical, psychological, and social health and thereby require special care and attention. Along with aging, older people experience declining functional status and are likely to have multiple chronic illnesses and mental health problems (Aday, 2000). This chapter aims to provide an overview of the gerontological mental health scenario in India with respect to mental health policies and services. Broadly, it deals with old age psychiatry in India, epidemiology of mental health problems, and mental health service requirements, integration and training.

OLD AGE PSYCHIATRY IN INDIA

India has bred a number of religious sects at different stages of its civilization and also adopted some alien religions and cultures. Over the past several decades of independent India, the lifestyle has become more complex under the shadows of various cults and cultures. In ancient India, people knew their specific roles and how they were to be performed during different stages of life, leaving little room for the development of psychogenic (exogenous) mental health problems. The burgeoning of the population to 1 billion, increasing life span, and the breakup of the traditional extended family have all contributed to the need to reform the geriatric services in India (Thara et al., 2004). It is estimated that there are already about 1.5 million people affected by dementia in India and this number is likely to increase in the coming decades (Feeri et al., 2005). The number of people affected by depression and other mental health problems is expected to surpass the number of those affected by dementia (Rao and Shaji, 2007). The lack of priority accorded to the healthcare needs of the elderly seems to perpetuate the low level of public awareness about mental health problems in old age. Dementia and other mental disorders of older people remain hidden, and are rarely brought to the attention of health care professionals and policy makers. There are hardly any specialized services for older people in the government run public healthcare services in India compared to other specialties. General health services remain clinic or hospital-based and typically involve long waits in crowded clinics/hospitals even for brief consultations. Trained health care workers play a pivotal role in providing outreach services in rural areas. However, they do not consider the care of older people their priority, instead prioritizing maternal and childcare (Rao and Shaji, 2007).

EPIDEMIOLOGY AND PROFILE OF MENTAL HEALTH PROBLEMS OF OLDER PERSONS

Older adults are considered to be an extension of the adult population and epidemiological studies focusing on older adults specifically are scarce in India. Reports of various epidemiological studies indicate a variable degree of mental health morbidity in older adults (10-16%). In Pondicherry (South India), psychiatric disorders among older adults were found to be 17.4% (Premarajan et al., 1993). Another epidemiological study from Uttar Pradesh (North India) reported 43.3% of the elderly to be suffering from one or the other mental health problems compared to 4.7% adults (Tiwari, 2000). Depression was three times more common than mania, occurring for the first time after 60 years (Rao, 1997). Depression was found to be a common diagnosis in the geriatric population (Tiwari et al., 2010). Studies from hospital clinics, community as well as old age homes found depression as the most common psychiatric disorder in the geriatric population with prevalence ranging from 22.2% to 55.2% of gero-psychiatric patients (Tiple et al., 2006; Rajkumar et al., 2009; Suresh Kumar et al., 2012). Suicide, especially due to depression, occurs more frequently in the elderly and adds to this problem (Rao and Madhavan, 1983). The prevalence of neurotic depression in the rural elderly was found to be 13.5%. A recent report indicates that 5.8% of the urban and 7.2% of the rural older adults primarily suffer from mood (affective) disorders; 2.4% of the urban and 2.1% of the rural older adults are primarily suffering from neurotic, stress-related and somatoform disorders; and 0.6% of urban and rural older adults primarily suffer from psychotic disorders (Tiwari and Pandey, 2012). The burden of mental health problems has been calculated on the basis of a recent study carried out in the country. The average prevalence of mental health problems both in rural and urban communities indicates that 20.5% of older adults are suffering from one or the other problems. Thus, 17.1 million older adults are suffering from one or the other diagnosable mental health problems in India (Tiwari and Pandey, 2012).

PREVALENCE OF MENTAL HEALTH PROBLEMS IN OLDER ADULTS IN INDIA

Like in many countries, older Indians are at an increased risk of developing some mental illnesses. Among these, depression and dementia seem to be the most common, however they are inadequately addressed. Suicide is also high in the older populations and often those who complete suicide also have a history of mental illness. The following table provides some data on the prevalence of cognitive disorders among older Indians, as well as co-morbidities.

Table 1. Prevalence of Mental Health Problems in Older Adults and their estimated number in India

Disorder category	Prevalence of mental health problems in urban older adults (per 1000)	Prevalence of mental health problems in rural older adults (per 1000)	Average prevalence of mental health problems in older adults [(U+R)÷2] (per 1000)	Estimated number (in million) of older adults suffering from mental health problems in India total older adults= 83.58
Psychiatric disorders other than cognitive disorders				
Without physical co-morbidity	31	77	54	4.51
With physical co-morbidity	66	82	74	6.18
Total	97	159	128	10.69
Cognitive disorders				
Without physical co-morbidity	18	27	23	1.92
With physical co-morbidity	38	39	39	3.26
Total	56	66	62	5.18
Both functional and cognitive disorders in the same subjects				
Without physical co-morbidity	04	06	05	0.42
With physical co-morbidity	16	05	11	0.92
Total	20	11	16	1.34
Dementia	44	28	3 6	3.01
Mild cognitive impairment	32	51	42	3.51
Total psychiatric morbidity				
Without physical co-morbidity	53	110	82	6.85
With physical co-morbidity	120	126	123	10.28
Total	173	236	205	17.13

Source: Tiwari and Pandey (2012).

Depression

Studies from hospital clinics, community as well as old age homes found depression to be the most common psychiatric disorder in the geriatric population with prevalence ranging from 22.2% to 55.2% of gero-psychiatric patients (Seby et al., 2011; Tiple et al., 2006; Rajkumar et al., 2009). Another study on the elderly population, in the community, inpatient, outpatient and old age homes have shown that depression is the most common mental illness in older people (Nandi et al., 1997; Tiwari, 2000; Chhabra and Kar, 2002). Nandi et al. (1997) studied psychiatric morbidity of the elderly population of a rural community in West Bengal. In a sample of 183 subjects (85 male, 98 female) they found 60% of the population to be mentally ill with higher morbidity among women (77.6%) than men (42.4%). There was significantly higher morbidity in the age group 70-74 compared to normal population. The total mental morbidity rate was as high as 612/1000 population. Depression was the most common illness of old age in this sample, the rate being 522/1000 population (101 cases out of 112 were diagnosed as cases of depression). Women presented a higher rate of depression (704/1000 population). An epidemiological study from rural Uttar Pradesh showed that psychiatric morbidity in the geriatric group (43.32%) was higher than in the non-geriatric group (4.66%) and the most common psychiatric morbidity was neurotic depression, followed by manic-depressive psychosis with depression and anxiety states. Psychiatric morbidity was more prevalent in those older persons who were socially, economically, and educationally disadvantaged (Tiwari, 2000).

Dementia

Dementia is an 'umbrella' term used to describe a collection of symptoms associated with physical changes in the brain that result in the gradual loss of mental functions such as memory and the ability to use words or to carry out previously familiar tasks. Dementia is defined as a syndrome of acquired impairment of memory and other cognitive functions secondary to structural brain damage (Moroney et al., 1997). The mental disorders frequently encountered in the Indian elderly include dementia and mood disorders in particular (Prakash and Kukreti, 2013). Dementia seems to be the silent epidemic next to depression among Indian elders. The prevalence of dementia in Indian studies has been shown to vary from 0.84% to 6.7% (Shaji et al., 2005; Prasad et al., 2009; Prince, 2009). Diabetes, depression, hyperlipidaemia, urban living, and lack of exercise are independent risk factors for dementia. Living in joint families and increased intake of polyunsaturated fats conferred protection against dementia (Tripathi et al., 2012).

Anxiety

Anxiety disorders are a common psychiatric problem in later life, affecting 3 to 15% of older adults (Bryant et al., 2008). Anxiety is considered excessive or pathological when it arises in the absence of challenge or stress, when it is out of proportion to the challenge or stress in duration or severity, when it results in significant distress, and when it results in psychological, social, occupational, biological, and other impairment (Trivedi and Gupta, 2010). The high rate of co-morbidity between late-onset generalized anxiety disorder and depression in old age suggests that antidepressant medication should be the treatment of choice (Flint, 1997). According to Trivedi and Gupta (2010) epidemiological data of anxiety disorder in special Indian populations like the elderly are scant. Further, in general, the status of anxiety disorder research from India in relation to epidemiology, phenomenology, course, outcome and management is lacking.

Suicide

Depression and suicide are probably the mental disorders most related to environmental, family, social, and religious factors (Thara et al., 2004). Elderly people have a higher risk of completed suicide than any other age group worldwide (WHO, 2002). Despite this, suicide in elderly people receives relatively little attention, with public health measures, medical research, and media attention focusing on younger age groups (Uncapher et al., 2000). According to psychological autopsy studies of suicides in elderly people, 71-95% of the people have had a major psychiatric disorder by the time of death (Conwell et al., 2002). Depressive illnesses are by far the most common and important diagnoses. In the only prospective, non-clinical cohort study of older people to date in which completed suicide was the outcome, self-rated severity of depressive symptoms was the strongest predictor of suicide (Ross et al., 1990). It is predicted that in the coming decades, there will be a tremendous increase in the number of elderly in India, with a similar increase in elderly suicide. Risk factors may co-occur leading to greater risk, such as social isolation and depression or depression and drug abuse. The suicidal behavior among the elderly, women, and adolescents are different from the other age groups or middle aged men (Rohit et al., 2007). Suicide is more likely to be missed in the elderly due to their indirect methods of communication regarding their suicidal intent (Garg et al., 2007). Suicide rates among the elderly (mean age 67.7) in South India, were reported to be 189/100,000 with the male female ratio being 1: 0.66 (Abraham et al., 2005).

MENTAL HEALTH SERVICE REQUIREMENTS FOR OLDER ADULTS IN INDIA

The professional and physical infrastructure requirements to serve mentally ill older adults have been worked out on the basis of norms as provided in the Mental Health ACT, 1987. The estimate of professional requirements have been worked out assuming that, of the total mentally ill older adults, about 50% (8.56 million) might be seeking professional help and, of these, only 7–10% (0.59–0.86 million) will be in need of psychiatric hospitalization. The requirements have been calculated taking an average of 8.5% (0.72 million) of patients who are in of need of hospitalization (Desai and Nambi, 2014). India has limited numbers of mental health professionals, with approximately 4000 psychiatrists catering to the 21 million people comprising the geriatric population in need of mental health services (Thirunavukarasu and Thirunavukarasu, 2010).

Table 2. Requirements (full figures) for geriatric mental health beds and manpower as per the mental Health Act, 1987, norms

Beds and manpower requirements	Mental Health Act, 1987, norms as modified by the Gazette of India no. 252	Estimated beds and manpower requirements
Beds	–	7,20,000
Qualified psychiatrists	1:100	7,200
Mental health professional assistant (clinical), psychologist or psychiatric social worker	1:100	7,200
Qualified medical officer (MBBS)	1:50	14,400
Staff nurse	1:10	72,000
Attendants	1:5	1,44,000

Table 3. Manpower norms and requirements for the general population vis-à-vis for older adults and the proposed estimates

Manpower requirement norms for the general population (Desai, 2004)	Manpower requirements for the general population – 1114.7 Millions	Manpower requirements for the elderly population – 83.58 Millions, as per the norms for the general population	Estimated geriatric mental health manpower requirements for the elderly (Five-times more than the general population)*
Psychiatrists (1 per 50,000 population)	0.022 (22,294)	0.0016 (1,672)	0.0083 (8,360)
Clinical psychologists (1 per 25,000 population)	0.044 (44,588)	0.0033 (3,343)	0.01 (17,715)
Psychiatric social workers (1 per 25,000 population)	0.044 (44,588)	0.0033 (3,343)	0.017 (17,715)
Psychiatric nurses (1 per 25,000 population)	0.044 (44,588)	0.0033 (3,343)	0.017 (17,715)

Source: Tiwari and Pandey (2012).

At present, most of the geriatric outpatient department (OPD) services are available only in tertiary care hospitals in big cities. Public sector hospitals suffer from problems of inaccessibility, inequitable distribution, lack of staff, drugs, and equipment while the private sector is largely unregulated with serious complaints regarding poor quality of care and unethical behaviour of professionals and staff (Biswas, 1994). Healthcare utilization is irregular across the country. It is found to be greater among older adults with higher levels of education, those living in urban areas and among those seeking treatment for communicable rather than non-communicable diseases (Prakesh and Prerna, 2013).

Caregiving

India has four types of resources to address geriatric mental health issues: 1) state funded psychiatric hospitals and nursing homes; 2) private psychiatric hospitals and nursing homes; 3) non-governmental organizations; and 4) the most important informal resource – familial caregivers. The country has limited numbers of mental health professionals, with around 4000 psychiatrists catering to the 21 million older persons in need of mental health services (Thirunavukarasu and Thirunavukarasu, 2010). In terms of infrastructure, very few Indian hospitals have geriatric units and most elderly patients are treated in general medical/ psychiatric wards. Further, the health insurance sector in India does not cover mental illness (Biswas, 1994). A large proportion of the population is forced to bypass free public services to pay out of pocket in private institutions (Shaji et al., 2010). In India, though new initiatives such as day care centres, old age residential homes, memory clinics, help lines, counseling, and recreational facilities are being developed, most of them are urban based. Non-governmental organizations like Help Age India, the Age Well Foundation, and the Dignity Foundation are actively contributing, but still efforts are far from reaching to the masses (Krishnaswamy et al., 2008).

The silver lining of clouds surrounding meagre geriatric mental health resources is undoubtedly the support of families, who, irrespective of their financial status, deem it their responsibility to care for their elderly mentally ill relatives. In the current era of modernization, globalization and changing social values, there is an apparent weakening of joint family systems. The traditional sense of filial piety, duty, and obligation of the younger generation towards their older generation is changing. The Indian elderly generation is caught between the decline in traditional values on the one hand and the absence of an adequate social security system, on the other (Bhat and Raj, 2001). The above factors have led to increased incidence of the elderly being abandoned by family members thus becoming homeless. State provided facilities such as day care centres and respite care are scarce. There is a sheer absence of any home based rehabilitation measures, domiciliary services, support services, or benefits accorded by the state to families to address care- givers' burden (Gupta, 2009). In terms of professional training and research, there are few opportunities for geriatric knowledge building and formal training in India.

Services and Professional Training

In terms of training professionals and conducting research, there are few opportunities for geriatric psychiatry knowledge building in India. Geriatric psychiatry is a neglected branch among the medical specialties. The Medical Council of India, the medical education regulatory body, offers this super specialty training only in very few places like Lucknow and Bangalore (Prakesh and Kukreti, 2013). Advocacy and research activities are only left to a few organizations like the Indian Association for Geriatric Mental Health, Geriatric Society of India, India Academy of Geriatrics, and the Association of Gerontologists (Gupta, 2009). In order to promote better mental health care for the older persons, primary health care providers (medical and paramedical) will have to be trained in the skills of geriatric mental health care (Tiwari and Pandey, 2012). At present, there is a need to expand the teaching curriculum across all the disciplines to include geriatric care components in graduate and post graduate medicine, psychiatric nursing, and psychiatric social work. Further, gerontological social work education can be offered by both central and state run institutions to meet the needs of the older population. There is a need to increase the seats in geriatric medicine specialty and geriatric psychiatry super specialty courses and to develop programmes to train general physicians and health workers to perform screening and make relevant referrals (Prakesh and Kukreti, 2013).

Indigenous Models of Intervention

Yoga-based intervention appears to have a beneficial effect on cognitive functions like delayed recall of verbal and visual memory, attention, executive function, and psychomotor speed when practiced for 6 months in the elderly. Additionally, Yoga-based intervention also appears beneficial in improving several domains of cognitive function among the elderly living in residential care homes (Hariprasad et al., 2013). Older persons who have a higher level of spirituality and practice yoga showed significant improvement in physical and mental health, and overall quality of life (Ilango and Udhayakumar, 2012). Several indigenous systems of medicine also operate in India amidst the formal public and private systems and offer treatments which may be more accessible, affordable, or acceptable to the rural elderly (Prakesh and Kukreti, 2013). Furthermore, a recent study suggests that graduates of indigenous medical programs often lack clinical training required to utilize diagnostic tools, conduct basic procedures, and handle primary care emergencies which has implications for older persons (Patwardhan et al., 2011).

POLICIES AND PROGRAMMES

The well-being of senior citizens is mandated in the Constitution of India under Article 41: "The state shall, within the limit of its economic capacity and development, make effective provision for securing the right to public assistance in case of old age" (Krishnaswamy et al., 2008). The most recent effort is the National Programme for the Health Care of the Elderly (NPHCE), released in early 2011 in which social security provisions for pension, income tax benefits, provident fund, gratuity, and medical assistance have been strengthened. Focus is shifting more on capacity building by: (1) expanding infrastructure to include Regional Geriatric Centres in district hospitals and opening community-based geriatric clinics; (2) establishing specialized geriatric training programs and research institutes; and (3) utilizing mass media to educate the public. The programme also aims to promote strong inter-organizational linkages and referral mechanisms, as well as training and support for informal caregivers. The programme is being implemented in phases beginning with 100 districts in 21 of India's 28 states (Government of India, 2012). However, the National Policy on Older Persons (NPOP) in India is geared mainly towards welfare aspects, not towards addressing specific mental health issues (Malhotra and Singh, 2015). Hence, there is a need of a new policy framework under which various programmes for mental health of older persons can be initiated and facilitated.

GERONTOLOGICAL MENTAL HEALTH IN INDIA – THE WAY FORWARD

The cultural heritage of India is very rich and affects every facet of society. The diagnosis, management, course, and outcome of mental illnesses are, therefore, influenced by cultural factors (Chaturvedi, 1993). To understand mental health in old age, one should be aware of lifestyle aspects as well as being familiar with the ancient Indian perspective in addition to possessing clinical abilities (Tiwari and Pandey, 2012). Using indigenous models of intervention like yoga and spirituality appears to have a beneficial effect on mental health of the older persons (Ilango and Udhayakumar, 2012). To enhance the state of geriatric mental health services in India, the recommendations suggested by Prakesh and Kukreti (2013) are that awareness needs to be spread regarding mental health problems, specifically addressing the needs of the geriatric population and availability of services in this regard. The teaching curriculum should be expanded to include geriatric care components for individuals studying to become general physicians, psychiatrists, psychologists, psychiatric nurses and psychiatric social work professionals. Also, there is a need to increase the seats in the geriatric medical specialty and geriatric psychiatry super specialty courses and, and to develop programmes for sensitizing general physicians and health workers for screening and providing appropriate referrals to appropriate mental health services for older persons.

To deliver comprehensive care beyond hospitals in the community, it is crucial that day care centres, respite care facilities, half way homes, and old age homes be developed and expanded. Good quality epidemiological, health services, and gerontological social work research are needed to generate awareness, shape health and social policy, and encourage the development of better services for patients and their caregivers. The urgent need for mental health care for the rapidly growing population of elderly could be met by providing brief additional training for doctors working in primary care. Psychogeriatric services in the country should aim to empower families providing home based care. This could be done by enlarging the role of multipurpose health workers and social workers, training them to provide family and community interventions for elderly people with dementia and other mental health conditions (Thara et al., 2004). Despite various policies for older persons being in place, the reality is that they have not been implemented in their true sense. Most of the policies discuss social benefits, in general, for the elderly and there is a lack of real concern for geriatric mental health. Policy makers should not forget the role of caregivers and families, and should utilize research-based practices, while simultaneously ensuring that they receive adequate support from health professionals and the community (Prakesh and Kureti, 2013).

CONCLUSION

India is witnessing a steady increase in the older population. The elderly population is facing a huge burden of communicable and non-communicable diseases. The most common mental health problems among Indian older persons are depression, dementia and anxiety disorders. Considering the size of the older age population, the psychogeriatric services for them are inadequate. Healthcare utilization is irregular across the country where only older adults with a higher socio economic status and higher levels of education are utilizing it. Apart from weekly geriatric psychiatry out-patient clinics run by a few hospitals, there is no formal mental health services for the elderly in India. The most pressing need is to provide brief, additional training for doctors and other health professionals working in primary care. Efforts are required to make treatment accessible, available, and affordable at the community level. There is an urgent need to review, develop and implement national policies and programmes for promoting geriatric mental health.

REFERENCES

Aday, L. A. (2000). At risk in America: The health and health care needs of vulnerable populations in the United States (2nd ed.). San Francisco: Jossey-Bass.

Abraham, V. J., Abraham, S. and Jacob, K.S. (2005). Suicide in the elderly in Kaniyambadi block, Tamil Nadu, South India. *International Journal of Geriatric Psychiatry,* 10, 953-955.

Biswas, S. (1994). Implication of population and aging. In C. Ramachandra and B. Shah, (Eds.), *Public health implications of aging in India* (pp. 22- 35). New Delhi: Indian Council of Medical Research.

Bhat, A. K. and Raj D. (2001). Ageing in India: drifting intergenerational relations, challenges and options. *Ageing Society*, 21(5). 621–40.

Bryant, C., Jackson, H. and Ames, D. (2008): The prevalence of anxiety in older adults: methodological issues and a review of the literature. *Journal of Affect Disorders,* 109(3). 233-250.

Chaturvedi, S. K. (1993). Neurosis across cultures. *International Review of Psychiatry,* 5, 179-91.

Chhabra, V. and Kar, N. (2002). Geriatric patients in a psychiatric ward: A 10 year profile. *Indian Journal of Psychiatry*, 44, S47.

Chandramouli, C. (2011). Census of India 2011 - A story of Innovations. Press Information Bureau, Government of India. Retrieved from http://www.censusindia.gov.in.

Desai, N. G., Tiwari, S. C., Nambi, S., Shah, B., Singh, R. A. and Kumar, D. (2004). Urban mental health services in India: How complete or incomplete? *Indian Journal of Psychiatry*, 46,195-212.

Egede, L. E. and Ellis, C (2010). Diabetes and depression: Global perspectives. *Diabetes Research and Clinical Practice*, 87(3), 302–12.

Flint, A. J. (1997). Epidemiology and comorbidity of anxiety disorders in later life: Implications for treatment. *ClinNeurosci,* 4 (1), 31-36.

Ferri, C. P., Prince, M., Brayne C, Carol, B., Brodaty, H. and Fratiglioni, L. (2005). Global prevalence of dementia: A Delphi consensus study. *Lancet,* 366 (2), 112-117.

Guha, R. (1994). Morbidity related epidemiological determinants in Indian aged - an overview. In C. R. Ramachandran and B. Shah (Eds), *Public health implications of ageing in India.* New Delhi: Indian Council of Medical Research.

Gokhale, S. (2003). Towards a policy for aging in India. *J Aging Soc Policy,* 15, 213- 34.

Gupta, R. (2009). Systems perspective: understanding care giving of the elderly in India. *Health Care Women International,* 30(12), 1040–54.

Hariprasad, V. R., Koparde, V., Sivakumar, P. T., Varambally, S., Thirthalli, J. and Varghese, M.(2013). Randomized clinical trial of yoga-based intervention in residents from elderly homes: Effects on cognitive function. *Indian J Psychiatry*, 55, S357-63.

Ilango, P. and Udhayakumar, P. (2012). Spirituality, Stress and Wellbeing among the Elders Practicing Spirituality. *SamajaKaryadaHejjegalu,* 2(10), 37 -42.

Khan, R. L. (1971). Psychological aspects of aging. In I. Rossman (Ed.), *Clinical geriatric* (pp.107 -113). Philadelphia: J.B. Lippincott.

Krishnaswamy, B., Than Sein, U., Davison, M., Cherian, V., Kavita Venkataraman and Leslie Anand (2008). Ageing in India. *Ageing International Journal,*: 258–268.

Moroney, J. T., Bagiella, E., Desmond, D. W., Hachinski, V. C., Molsa,. P. K., Gustafson, L., Fischer, P. (1997). Meta-analysis of the Hachinski Ischiaemic Score in pathologically verified dementias. *Neurology*, 49(4), 96-105.

Moussavi, S., Chatterji, S., Verdes, E., Tandon, A., Patel, V. and Ustun, B. (2007). Depression, chronic diseases, and decrements in health: results from the World Health Surveys. *The Lancet,* 370, 851–58.

Malhotra, S. and Singh, A. (2015). Acute and Transient Psychosis: An overview. In S. Malhotra and S. Chakrabarthi (Eds.), *Developments in Psychiatry in India: Clinical, Research and Policy Perspectives* (pp.99-138). New Delhi: Springer.

Nandi, D. N., Ajmany, S., Ganguli, H., Banerjee, G., Boral, G.C. and Ghosh, A. (1976). The incidence of mental disorders in one year in a rural community in West Bengal. *Indian Journal of Psychiatry*, Vol.18: 79-87.

Nandi, P.S., Banerjee, G., Mukherjee, S.P., Nandi, S. and Nandi, D.N. (1997). A study of psychiatric morbidity of the elderly population of a rural community in West Bengal. *Indian Journal of Psychiatry*, 39(2), 122-129.

Premarajan, K. C., Danabalan, M., Chandrasekar, R. and Srinivasa, D. K. (1993). Prevalence of psychiatry morbidity in an urban community of Pondicherry. *Indian Journal of Psychiatry*, 35(2), 99-102.

Prasad, K., Gupta, H., Bharath, S., Prakash, O., Sivakumar,. P. T., Kumar, C. N. and Varghese, M. (2009). Clinical practice with antidementia and antipsychotic drugs: audit from a geriatric clinic in India. *Indian Journal Psychiatry,* 51(4), 27-25.

Prince, M. J. (2009). The 10/66 dementia research group - 10 years on. *Indian J Psychiatry,* 51(1), 8–15.

Patwardhan, K., Gehlot, S., Singh, G. and Rathore, H. C. (2011). The ayurveda education in India: how well are the graduates exposed to basic clinical skills? *Evid Complement Alternat Med.* doi: 10.1093/ecam/nep113.

Prakesh, O. and Prerna (2013). *State of Geriatric Mental Health in India*. The current translational geriatrics and expeimental gerontology reports, 2, 1-6.

Ramachandran, V. and Menon, M.S. (1979). Ramamurthy B. Psychiatric disorders in subjects aged over fifty. *Indian Journal Psychiatry*, 22, 193-198.

Ramachandran, V., MenonSarada, M. and Arunagiri, S. (1982). Socio-cultural factors in late onset depression. *Indian Journal Psychiatry*, 24, 268-73.

Rao, A.V. and Madhavan, T. (1983). Depression and suicide behaviour in theaged. *Indian Journal of Psychiatry*. 25, 251–9.

Ross, R. K., Bernstein, L., Trent, L., Henderson, B. E. and Paganini-Hill, A. (1990). A prospective study of risk factors for traumatic death in the retirement community. *Preventive Medicine*, 19(3), 323-324.

Rao, A.V. (1997). Psychiatric morbidity in the aged. *Indian Journal of Medical Research*, 106, 361-369.

Rohit, G., Trivedi, J. K. and Mohen, D. (2007). Suicidal Behaviour in Special Population: Elderly, Women and Adolescence in Reference to India. *Delhi Psychiatric Journal,* 1(2), 106 -117.

Rajkumar, A. P., Thangadurai, P., Senthilkuma, P., Gayathri, K., Prince, M. and Jacob, K. S. (2009). Nature, prevalence and factors associated with depression among the elderly in a rural south Indian community. *International Psychogeriatric*, 21(2), 372–378.

Rao, T. S. and Shaji, K. S. (2007). Demographic aging: Implications for mental health. *Indian Journal of Psychiatry*, 49(2), 78-80.

Rajkumar, A. P., Thangadurai, P., Senthilkuma, P., Gayathri, K., Prince, M. and Jacob, K. S. (2009). Nature, prevalence and factors associated with depression among the elderly in a rural south Indian community. *International Psychogeriatric*, 21(2), 372–8.

Reddy, M.V. and Chandrashekhar, C.R. (1998). Prevalence of Mental and Behavioural Disorders in India: A meta- analysis. *Indian Journal of Psychiatry,* 40, 149-51.

RohitGarg, Trivedi, J. K. and MohanDhyani (2007). Suicidal Behaviour in Special Population: Elderly, Women and Adolescent in Special Reference to India. *Delhi Psychiatric Journal*, 10(2), 106- 118.

Shaji, S., Bose, S. and Kuriakose, S. (2009). Behavioral and psychological symptoms of dementia: A study of symptomatology. *Indian Journal of Psychiatry,* 51, 38-41.

Shaji, K. S., Iype, T. and Praveenlal, K. (2009). Dementia clinic in general hospital settings. *Indian Journal of Psychiatry,* 51, 42-44.

Shaji, K. S, Jithu, V. P. andJyothi, K. S. (2010). Indian research on aging and dementia. *Indian Journal of Psychiatry*, 52, 148-52.

Shaji, K. S., George, R. K., Prince, M. J. and Jacob, K. S.(2009). Behavioral symptoms and caregiver burden in dementia. *Indian Journal of Psychiatry*, 51, 45-49.

Shaji, S., Bose, S. and Varghese, A. (2005). Prevalence of dementia in an urban population in Kerala, India. *British Journal of Psychiatry*. 186, 136–40.

Shankardass and Kapur, M. (1995). Towards the Welfare of the Elderly in India. *Bold*, 5(4), 25-29.

Schneider, F. and Grozinger, M. (2010). Psychiatric illness through the lifespan. *European Archives of Psychiatry and Clinical Neuroscience*, 260 (2), 79–80.

Seby, K., Chaudhury, S. and Chakraborty, R. (2011). Prevalence of psychiatricand physical morbidity in an urban geriatric population. Indian *Journal of Psychiatry*. 53(2), 121–127.

Sureshkumar, R., Bharath, S., Jain, S., Prakash, O., Purushottam, M., Thennarasu, K., Varghese, M. (2012). ApoE4 and late onset depression in Indian population. *Journal of Affect Disorders*, 136(3), 244–248.

Tiwari, S. C. (2000). Geriatric Psychiatric Morbidity in Rural Northern India: Implications for the Future. *International Psychogeriatric*, 12, 35-48.

Travedi, J. K. (2000). Psychological Manifestations of Aging. *Indian Journal of Psychiatry*, 42(3), 223-224.

Tiple, P., Sharma, S. N. and Srivastava, A. S. (2006). Psychiatric morbidity in geriatric people. *Indian Journal of Psychiatry,* 48(2), 88–94.

Trivedi, J. K. and Gupta, P. K. (2010). An overview of Indian research in anxiety disorders. *Indian Journal of Psychiatry*, 52 (7), 210-218.

Thirunavukarasu, M. A and Thirunavukarasu, P. (2010). Training and National deficit of psychiatrists in India - a critical analysis. *Indian Journal of Psychiatry,* 52 (7), 83–88.

Tiwari, S. C., Singh, R., Kohli, V. K. and Agarwal, G. G. (2010). An epidemiological study of prevalence of neuro-psychiatric disorders with special reference to cognitive disorders, amongst (rural) elderly- Lucknow study. New Delhi: ICMR Report.

Tripathi, M., Vibha, D., Gupta, P., Bhatia, R., Srivastava, M. V., Vivekanandhan, S., Mendez, M. F. (2012). Risk factors of dementia in North India: a case– control study. *Aging Mental Health*, 16(2), 228–35.

Tiwari, S. C, Pandey, N. M. and Singh, I. (2012). Mental health problems among inhabitants of old age homes: A preliminary study. *Indian Journal Psychiatry,* 54(2), 144-148.

Tiwari, S. C. and Pandey, N. M. (2013). The Indian concepts of lifestyle and mental health in old age. *Indian J Psychiatry*, 55 (6), 288-292.

Uncapher, H. and Arean, P. A. (2000). Physicians are less willing to treat suicidal ideation in older patients. *Journal of American Geriatric Society*, 48, 188-192.

UN population Division (2001). World population prospects, the 2000 revision. New York: United Nations publication.

United Nations (2002). *World population ageing: 1950–2050.* New York: Department of Economic and Social Affairs, Population Division: United Nations.

United Nations (2011). World Urbanization Prospects: The 2011 Revision Highlights. United Nations, Department of Economic and Social Affairs/Population Division. United Nations, New York. Retrieved from http://esa.un.org/unup/pdf/WUP2011_Highlights.pdf.

Waern, M. (2003). Alcohol dependence and alcohol misuse in elderly suicides. Alcohol and Alcoholism, 38(3), 249-254.

Wang, H. S. and Busse, E. W. (1971). Dementia in old age. In C.E. Wells (Ed.), *Dementia* (pp. 152-162). Philadelphia, PA: F.A. Davis.

WHO (2001). World Health Report: Mental Health: New understanding New Hope. Geneva.

WHO (2003). Investigating in Mental Health – A Report. Department of Mental Health and Substance Dependence, Non-communicable Diseases and Mental Health, World Health Organization, Geneva.

WHO (2005). *Promoting mental health: Concepts, emerging evidence, practice.* Geneva: WHO.

Wig, N. N. (2001). World Health Day. *Indian Journal of Psychiatry*, 43(1), 1-4.

PART III: LOW HUMAN DEVELOPMENT COUNTRIES

In: Ageing and Mental Health: Global Perspectives
Editors: Wendy Wen Li, Sherry M. Cummings et al.
ISBN: 978-1-63484-777-3

Chapter 12

OLD AGE MENTAL HEALTH IN UGANDA

Betty Kyaddondo*
National Population Council - Uganda

ABSTRACT

Uganda's life expectancy has tremendously improved in recent years, with 4.7% of the population aged over 60 years. Despite the policy reforms within the ministry of health, including creating a department of the elderly and the disabled in the Ministry of Gender, a lot still remains to be done. Social security benefits are not only very small, but most elderly people are too weak to perform productive work and are economically dependent on others like their children, grandchildren, relatives, and neighbours for survival. Increasing numbers of the elderly even bear the burden of looking after their grandchildren with their meager resources due to death of the parents of the children, mostly from HIV/AIDS.

As people age, their healthcare needs generally increase, but there are inadequate systems in place to keep track of the health trend of older people, and society is not yet coping with the provision of appropriate services. Failing health and rising expenses are a major source of worry and stress among the elderly. Older people are currently finding huge barriers to accessing healthcare and the elderly with mental health disorders have not been given the appropriate attention. Many of those elderly with mental illnesses may not even report for health care services.

Keywords: elderly, mental health, ageing, gerontology, HIV/AIDS

INTRODUCTION

As per the 2002 Census, only 5% of Uganda's 24.2 million people were aged 60 years and above, while 50% were less than 15 years. This is compared to 4.1% during the 1991 Census. As is the situation worldwide, the elderly population in Uganda is therefore growing fast. At an annual rate of 7.4%, the ageing population in Uganda will double to 3 million in

* Corresponding author: Betty Kyaddondo, National Population Council - Uganda. Email: bettykyad@gmail.com.

less than 10 years (Uganda Reach the Aged Association, 2009). The Uganda National House Hold Survey Report of 2009/2010 indicated that the population of older persons in Uganda was 1,304,464 of which 703,811 were females. The 2012/13 Uganda National Household Survey on the other hand, indicated a total of 1,580,261 older persons (UBOS 2014). In 2013, the Uganda Bureau of Statistics estimated that the total population of Uganda was at 34.5 million and the proportions of older persons have not changed much (UBOS 2014).

The Government of the Republic of Uganda comprehensively developed the National Policy for Older Persons in 2009 with guidance and support of many stakeholders, coordinated through the Ministry of Gender, Labor and Social Development (MGLSD, 2009). The Policy provides a framework for addressing, programming and legislation to identify opportunities and harness the potential of older persons. Subsequently, the National Minimum Health Care Package exists but pays little attention to the specific needs of the older people (WHO SAGE-Uganda, 2011).

The HIV/AIDS scourge had a major toll on the well being of the elderly in Uganda. Many of these older people have lost family to HIV/AIDS, meaning they can't rely on traditional family support as they get older and will often be required to look after grandchildren following the death of parents. Around half of Ugandan orphans are looked after by grandparents (Katie Chronicles, 2010).

There is scanty information about the mental health of the elderly in Uganda, mainly because the special medical problems of the elderly are not addressed by the health care system, yet most illnesses for the elderly are treated on non-psychiatric wards (Nakasujja Noeline et al., 2007) with possibility of missing or misdiagnosing the psychiatric elderly patients (Ruegg et al., 1988).

Culture and Context of Older Persons in Uganda

In traditional Ugandan society, older persons were revered and respected for their wisdom and experience (Uganda Reach the Aged Association, 2009). Their counsel was sought in times of crisis and their decision was final. Older people were also the vehicles through which traditional customs and values were passed from one generation to another. Social gatherings could not even be held without the presence of older persons. Today, those traditions have been largely discarded, and there is evidence that Uganda's older persons do not enjoy the privileged position they once were assured (Cohen and Menken, 2006). Although they still play an important role in society, they are not acknowledged. The prevailing negative attitude towards the elderly leads to suffering for this group (Kabole, 2003), predisposing them to psychiatric illnesses.

Across the continent, millions of families would not survive without the contribution of older people – from caring for orphaned grandchildren and infected own children to providing much needed household income (HelpAge International, 2008). Older persons in Uganda contribute immensely to the creation of wealth, support and care for children including HIV/AIDS orphans, creation of social cohesion and conflict resolution in their communities and the nation as a whole (MOGLSD, 2009). They make valuable contributions to society as guardians of traditions and cultural values that are passed on from generation to generation

(Cummings and Galambous, 2005). Today, the African traditional forms of caring for older people are changing.

Like in most parts of Africa, Uganda is not excepted from some forms of violence against older women which is based on cultural practices that specifically target widows who are regarded as insignificant without their husbands. While widows of all ages are subjected to mistreatment, older widows are particularly vulnerable because age lowers their status in the community and makes caring for them more difficult. Older women face double tragedy in this regard, and are increasingly abused physically, socially, economically, and psychologically by their families and/or communities. They are segregated and marginalised leading to loneliness, loss of self-esteem, and economic deprivation (Golaz and Rutaremwa, 2011). Some older women are abused sexually and physically, aggravating their vulnerability to mental health concerns. Socio-economic changes in the country have weakened family structure, denying older persons adequate care and provision. Family bonds have been weakened by the high cost of living, HIV/AIDS, and urbanisation, which have led families to live far from villages where many older persons still reside. Most people have little understanding of mental disorders and do not know that effective treatments and services are available. Like elsewhere in developing countries, most mentally ill patients, including the elderly, seek care from traditional healers (Kapur, 2007), and only end up at the health facilities as a last resort.

The Impact of HIV/AIDS

The role of grandparents in the care of children has been emphasised (Cattell Maria, 1990 and Zimmer Zachary, 2005). In Uganda, it is estimated that 50% of double orphans (those who are without a mother and father) are cared for by older people. Despite this, older people are often excluded from development programmes and discriminated against by health care and other services. Despite their indispensable contribution, many older people in Africa continue to experience deepening poverty, discrimination, violence, and abuse (HelpAge International, 2009), and are unable to access benefits to which they should be entitled.

Globally, older people are sexually active and at risk of HIV infection (Cooperman, 2007). This, compounded with the fact that Ugandan older people are caring for others who have been affected by HIV/AIDS, further exacerbates the difficulty of their situation. The care role aggravates their poverty, while putting them at risk of infection from direct contact with sick relatives. AIDS claims the lives of younger family members who older people would otherwise depend upon for support. With an estimated 1.7 million orphans, Uganda has the highest proportion of AIDS orphans in the whole world (Ntozi and Ahimisibwe, 2011).

Older people are also more likely to have co-morbidities, more likely to experience a rapid progression to AIDS and, consequently, to have lower survival rates. There is also increased risk of side effects from anti retroviral therapy (ART; used in the management of HIV/AIDS)and an elevated risk of psychiatric disorders (Llorente and Malphurs, 2006). The Uganda AIDS Indicator Survey 2004 – 05 showed that HIV prevalence among older people is lower than in people under 5, but only slightly so (Ministry of Health, 2006).

Socio Economic Profile

Studies have singled out the older population as prone to poverty. Older people in Uganda perceive old age as characterised by ill-health, dependency, low income and depreciated asset bases, changed body features, and changed physiological state (Najjumba-Mulindwa, 2003). Najjumba-Mulindwa (2003) further found that the single, widowed, disabled, women and the elderly living alone are most prone to chronic poverty resulting from unemployment, chronic ill health, lack of skills, HIV/AIDS, lack of social security systems, low land productivity, political instability, low agricultural returns, and functional inability due to old age, which predisposes them to mental stress and depression.

Many older people in Uganda live in rural areas, where there are fewer social services (Population Secretariat, 2013). They experience economic exclusion, and are often denied employment and access to insurance or credit schemes. Pensions are rare and mainly concern former civil servants. In Uganda, as in many African societies, when older persons living alone need help, a common practice is to entrust them to one of their grandchildren (Golaz and Rutaremwa, 2011). The child takes care of his or her grandparent while maintaining the link between the household of origin and that of the elderly person. But, conversely, an elderly person cannot refuse the custody of a child (Williams, 2003), to the extent that some older people find themselves with several dependent children in their care. This role is sometimes imposed upon older adults (Seeley et al., 2009) but the presence of a child within the household often also provides a source of help for an elderly person (Ssengonzi, (2007). An older adult living with a child is relatively less vulnerable than a person living alone, because in addition to the help that he or she brings, the child provides access to wider family support. However the child might be a socio-economic burden to the older person in need of care as children themselves require care.

The majority of older persons live in semi-permanent or makeshift structures, usually grass thatched with mud walls; the homeless elderly move from place to place, sometimes occupying abandoned structures (Golaz and Rutaremwa, 2011). The dilapidated state of the houses they occupy puts them and their dependants in danger as they threaten to collapse over them, especially during the rains. The walls, floors, and roofs are full of cracks, exposing them to cold and harmful animals and insects. Some of the diseases that the elderly suffer from are related to the poor conditions they live in. Lack of personal effects such as bedding and adequate clothing aggravates the health problem, including mental illnesses. Older persons depend on one meal a day; others survive on a meal for two or more days. Usually this is one type of food only (Kikafunda and Lukwago, 2005). Lack of a balanced diet leaves many emaciated and exposed to diseases that could be avoided. Malnutrition remains another health problem among older people, especially those living in rural areas. Research also revealed that lack of clean water is another crucial problem for older persons in Uganda (Uganda Reach the Aged Association, 2009). Older adults are forced to travel long distances to find clean water. Dependence on contaminated water puts their health at risk.

Access to Health and Related Care

Similar to the scarcity of reliable population-based information about disease, disability and health risks in the older population, there is limited data about geriatric service provision and utilisation in Uganda. There is not enough research, but through many media reports, it is clear that transforming health care has not all been positive for poor and older citizens and, in particular, has resulted in the marginalisation of geriatric services in Uganda.

According to the 2013 World Population Ageing Report, the most common problems among older people include visual impairment, cancer, hypertension, diabetes, osteoporosis, dementia, and depression (United Nations, 2013). Older people are usually more susceptible to fatal forms of malaria owing to age-associated loss of immune function (Herrmann and Krause, 2004). Health care is, however, inaccessible to older people due to high cost and long distances to medical services. With the country's patchy and complex healthcare system, many elderly people with multiple health needs shun health units, overwhelmed by the long waits and complicated procedures. There is no doubt that there is limited information on the health and wellbeing of older persons (WHO SAGE, 2011). In Uganda in particular, older adults have lesser access to health facilities than others, and there are few adapted health facilities (Najjumba 2003). Failure to tackle the old age vulnerability especially in terms of access to health services equates to a failure to fulfill basic human rights.

Despite the above conditions, it is a distressing reality that the use of gerontology inpatient and outpatient health services in Uganda is far below par. Given such vulnerability to many diseases and health conditions, there are numerous factors accounting for this apparent state of apathy towards the unmet health as well as mental health needs of the elderly. There are some obvious health and social care policy gaps at the macro level. The government's historical priorities have been maternal and child health and this may not be easy to change quickly or easily in terms of policies targeted at older people. Additionally, there is a mentality that older people are less productive than young people and therefore, less deserving of healthcare. This has exacerbated the effects of ageing in a country that already has a weak and under-developed health system.

Mental Health Care and the Elderly

Poor mental health can engender poor physical health and vice versa (Peters S 2003). The Ugandan government recognises mental health as a serious public health and development concern, and has recently implemented a number of reforms aimed at strengthening the country's mental health system (Fred Kigozi et al., 2010). Some hope generally exists for better mental health programmes.

The devolution of mental health was stimulated in 1996, when the World Health Organisation (WHO) encouraged the Ministry of Health to strengthen mental health services and integrate them into primary health care (Kigozi, 2007). Standards and guidelines were developed for the care of children and adults with epilepsy and other mental disorders from community level to tertiary institutions. Health workers were trained to recognise and manage or refer common mental and neurological disorders. A new referral system was established along with a supervisory support network. Linkages were set up with other programmes such as for those with HIV/AIDS and health education for adolescents.

In order to improve service utilisation and uptake, efforts were made to raise awareness of mental health in the general population. A draft Mental Health Policy was developed in 2000 (Kigozi et al., 2010). The Mental Health Act was revised and integrated into a Health Services Bill (Chris Kiwawulo, 2010). Since then, mental and neurological drugs have been included in the essential drugs list. At the same time, the ministry also equipped mental health units at 13 regional referral hospitals countrywide to help treat patients, a move that aimed at reducing the capacity of the 900-bed national psychiatric hospital in Butabika by at least half. According to the second Health Sector Strategic Plan 2005, mental health is now included as one of twelve components of the National Minimum Health Care Package to be provided at all levels of care (Ministry of Health [MOH], 2005).

Despite the reforms and subsequent improvement of mental health services, Uganda's mental health system still faces a number of shortcomings. Butabika hospital remains the only national referral mental hospital (MOH, 2010). There is a general lack of trained human resources and a scarcity of funding, with no special provisions for mental health funding (Flisher et al., 2009; Ndyanabangi, 2004). According to the 2006 WHO-AIMS assessment report, only 1% of health care expenditures by the Uganda government's ministry of health were specifically directed towards mental health in primary care. However, as part of the integrated health service delivery, other aspects of mental health are funded within the general health budget as well. The support from donors, including from the African Development Bank (ADB), raised the financial base to approximately 4% (Kigozi et al., 2010).

In 2011, Uganda had only 28 psychiatrists for a population of 33 million people and mental health units had very low numbers of medical professionals in the field of psychiatry. Most mental health service provision is done by clinical officers and nurses due to the inadequacy of mental health specialists. In addition, most medical students rarely opt for psychiatry because it is less lucrative. Not even scholarships can lure students to pursue psychiatry at post graduate level (Kiwawulo, 2010).

The WHO SAGE report 2011 revealed that many older people are lonely and feel depressed, calling for a need for service providers to add the component of psychosocial support as they deliver services to them. Despite this, in Uganda, many mentally ill elderly patients end up on non-psychiatric wards owing to somatisation of their illnesses (Noeline Nakasujja et al., 2007) and for some, a psychiatric diagnosis may be missed or misdiagnosed (Ruegg et al., 1988).

Mental health problems are increasing, with depression at 12-68%, anxiety disorders at 20-62% and alcohol dependency at 14% in the general population (MOH, 2007). According to one of the Consultant Psychiatrists at Butabika National referral hospital, depression and dementia are the most commonly diagnosed conditions among the elderly in Uganda. Data from supervision reports shows that about 75% of attendances at Mental Health Clinics have some form of neurological problem, commonly epilepsy, with cases of dementia on the rise, especially among persons living with HIV/AIDS.

In the attempt to assess prevalence of depression among HIV patients in the WHO SAGE study, 22 people (4.3%) were diagnosed with depression, the majority (28%) of whom were women, compared to only 16% of men. In the same vein, 48% of elderly in-patients in the study of psychiatric disorders (Nakasujja et al., 2007) were diagnosed with a psychiatric illness. Some of the predisposing factors to mental illness included: divorce/separation, low education levels, dependants within the household, and having no children offering support. Previous studies reported a similar profile of the elderly (Mugisha, 1985; Uganda MOFPED 1995a and 1995b). Post Traumatic Stress Disorder (PTSD) as a result of events that cause horror is the most common mental illness among people in Northern Uganda. This condition emerged in Uganda as a result of the 1987 to 2008 protracted Lord's Resistance Army war in which thousands of people were brutally killed (Kiwawulo 2010). Fortunately, the Consultant psychiatrist reported that mental illnesses are often treatable, although somewhat expensively. A patient with mental health problems is handled by many experts including doctors, counsellors, and psychologists, making the cost very high.

THE POLICY ENVIRONMENT

The Government of the Republic of Uganda has realised the increasing population of older persons and is committed to addressing their concerns (Kigozi 2010). It recognises that as people reach old age, they should continue enjoying dignified lives through active participation in economic, social, cultural, and political spheres as stipulated in the National Policy for Older Persons (MOGLSD, 2009). The government, therefore, is determined to enhance the recognition of the contributions of older persons and to eliminate all forms of neglect, abuse and violence against older persons.

The 1995 Constitution recognises the value and rights of the elderly. Article 32 of the constitution stipulates that: "The State shall make reasonable provision for the welfare and maintenance of the aged." Chapter 4 of Uganda's Constitution stipulates the rights and freedoms every Ugandan should enjoy, including the right to basics of life and a life of dignity. Article XIV of Uganda's Constitution (1995): states: "All Ugandans enjoy rights and opportunities and access to education, health services, decent shelter, adequate clothing, food security and pension and retirement benefits." Article 32 of the Constitution regarding affirmative action in favour of marginalised groups states that: "Not withstanding anything in the Constitution, the State shall take affirmative action in favor groups marginalized on the basis of sex, race, color, ethnic origin, tribe, creed, gender, age, or any other reason created by history, tradition or custom for the purpose of redressing imbalances which exist against them."

The Government is also a signatory to UN Conventions. The ILO Convention 102 of June 2001 sets out the minimum standards of social security benefits for old age, invalidity, survivors, medical care, sickness, unemployment, employment injury, family, and maternity benefits (International Labor Office, 2001). The Uganda Human Rights Commission, a body established under Article 51 of the Constitution of Uganda 1995, and the Uganda Human Rights Act No 4 1997, promote and protect human rights and investigate at its own initiative a violation of any human rights, including the rights of older persons (OHCHR, 2013).

The Ministry of Gender, Labour and Social Development, has a full-fledged Department of Disability and Elderly, with a Minister of State for Disability and Elderly Affairs. The Department is responsible for initiating policies, plans, laws and programs to protect and promote rights of older persons. For instance, there exists the rights-based National Policy for Older Persons (2009), the National Council for Older persons Act (2012) and the National

Plan of Action for older persons 2012/2013-2016/2017, which are all in line with the Madrid International Plan of Action on Ageing.

Regarding health care, Uganda developed a National Minimum Health Care Package and promoted Public-Private partnerships to ensure that people receive appropriate health services; but these initiatives have not paid the necessary attention to the specific health needs of older people (WHO SAGE, 2011). Mental health services in Uganda were decentralised in the 1960s and mental health units were built at regional referral hospitals. According to the WHO report on mental health policy and service provision 2010, the mental health units were managed by psychiatric clinical officers and had low staff morale, chronic shortage of drugs, and inadequate funds for community activities. Since the decentralisation of mental health services, the government of Uganda improved pre-service and in-service training for mental health workers with rehabilitation and remodelling of the mental health infrastructure in the country (Ndyanabangi et al., 2004). But the burden of mental disorders in Uganda is high in a country that is poorly resourced.

Caregiving and Social Support Systems

Traditionally, the Ugandan social structure was organised around the family and community. The African extended family network knitted together a network of blood relations, in-laws, and close friends (Kenneth, 2012). This network acted as insurance against all disabilities of old age and other shortcomings. The young and energetic were insurance for their older folks and took care of their needs. Sadly, several factors have interfered with the treasured network leaving the elderly vulnerable. While the traditional system has diminished, it has not been replaced by any other form of social security that caters to the elderly. Many older people, especially women, still find great satisfaction in providing care and support within their households, either to fellow adults or to children/grandchildren despite the difficulties of caregiving. Alternatively, older people need to be cared for, but it is often difficult to obtain the care. The few lucky ones receive care from their daughters, sons, or siblings in the form of financial assistance to pay for health care, medicine, schooling, food, and clothing (WHO SAGE 2011). Grandchildren in some instances provide physical assistance such as fetching water, agricultural work, cooking, and buying food. The burden of caregiving is manageable for the older people who receive the support they need from family, community and service providers, but if the conditions are not met, as may often be the case, caregiving of the elderly, becomes a burden that endangers their wellbeing.

There are some registered organisations that have emerged to assist older persons in many ways because they often lack a voice and, as already discussed, are often marginalised. Most of these organisations are community-based and are uncoordinated and poorly funded. Consequently, the impact of their activities and programmes has gone largely unnoticed. Moreover, older persons have just recently been included in National and Local Government structures; thus, their needs and concerns have, in the past, not been represented.

The Uganda Reach the Aged Association (URAA) was formed in 1991. The Association coordinates the activities of the aged care organisations in Uganda. It was established to tackle the problems of older people and to draw attention to their unique issues in order to create a lasting improvement in their lives. The URAA advocates for the improved quality of life and preservation of the dignity of older persons in Uganda (Uganda Reach the Aged Association, 2010).

The Child and Elderly Support Organization (CESO), an initiative that transforms the lives of children and elderly people who live under horrible and hard life conditions, focuses on giving education to vulnerable children and developing their talents, as well as supporting elderly care (CESO, 2013). More support is provided to the elderly in their homes especially if there are some caretakers in the homes. A few older people are under the care of the organisation, mainly those who don't have caretakers at home. CESO works to help the elderly socially, emotionally, financially, and in as many other ways possible so that they don't feel lonely, isolated, or neglected.

Joy For Elderly Care – Uganda is a charitable nongovernmental organisation that was founded in November 2006 to help the elderly, their children, and their grandchildren live a more meaningful and decent life. Currently located in the Kampala District, the organisation enables elderly persons to engage in small but productive businesses within their homes, such as markets, craft making, and small gardening to meet their financial needs and enable them to look after their grandchildren and any other vulnerable children within their care.

The Uganda Rural Elderly Support (URES) is a non-governmental organisation established in 2007 to assist the elderly in rural areas by enabling them to obtain skills and facilities for their livelihood (Uganda Rural Elderly Support, n.d.). The needy rural elderly vary from those staying alone with no relative to those with orphans and grandchildren. URES assists the elderly in Uganda to seek health care from Health Centres. At the health centres, the sick are treated and given drugs while URES meets the medical costs, since the elderly cannot pay for their medical bills.

HelpAge has worked in Uganda since the early 1990s with its the URAA and other partners. The two organisations focus on empowering older people to demand their rights and entitlementsm including benefiting from the existing national poverty reduction programmes in Northern Uganda. HelpAge's projects endeavour to encourage more effective health services as well as ensuring older people are included in key national health and HIV and AIDS programmes.

Coping Mechanisms for Caretakers

Many people with mental illness must rely on family and friends for support and to help them in their daily activities (World Federation for Mental Health [WFMH], 2014). Some patients with mental health problems may become aggressive, and caretakers are advised to accept their condition and have a positive attitude towards them (Kiwawulo, 2010). The caretakers of mental health patients need regular counselling, lest they develop psychological problems as well. It was also revealed by the WFMH that caring for those with neurological disorders requires tireless effort, energy, and empathy, and greatly impacts the daily lives of caregivers (WFMH, 2014). The caregivers must be educated on the fundamental aspects of mental health care, they should strive to make friends with the patients to avoid rejection, and most importantly, to make it easier for the caregiver to look after them.

Caretaking of the elderly is fast becoming a complex issue, worse still for family members of mentally ill elderly patients. Some caregivers instead of understanding the mental

Ministry of Health (2000). *Health Sector Strategic Plan I.* Retrieved from http://siteresources.worldbank.org/INTPRS1/Resources/383606-12018 83571938/Uganda_HSSP.pdfMinistry of Health (2005). *Health Sector Strategic Plan II.* Retrieved from http://siteresources.worldbank.org/INTPRS1/Resources/383606-1201883571938/Uganda_HSSP_2.pdf Ministry of Health (2010). *Health Sector Strategic Plan III.* Retrieved fromhttp://www.health.go.ug/docs/HSSP_III_2010.pdf.

Ministry of Health (2006). *Uganda-AIDS indicator survey 2004-2005, HIV/AIDS Sero-Behavioural Survey.* Retrieved from http://dhsprogram. com/pubs/pdf/ais2/ais2.pdf.

Nakasujja, N., Musisi, S., Walugembe, J. and Wallace,D. (2007). Psychiatric disorders among the elderly on non-psychiatric wards in an African setting. *International Psychogeriatrics Association, 19*, 1-14.

Najjumba-Mulindwa, I. (2003). *Chronic Poverty among the elderly in Uganda: perceptions, experiences and policy issues.* Prepared for Staying Poor: Chronic Poverty and Development Policy, University of Manchester, UK. Retrieved from http://docs.mak.ac.ug/sites/default/files/Chronic%20PovertyMulwinda.pdf.

Ndyanabangi S, Basangwa D, Lutakome J, Mubiru C (2004). Uganda mental health country profile. *International Review of Psychiatry*, 16(1-2), 54-62.

Ntozi, J. P. M. (1997). Effect of AIDS on children: the problem of orphans in Uganda. *Health transition review*, 7, 23–40.

Ntozi, J. P. and Ahimisibwe, F. (2001). Prospects for fertility decline in the face of HIV/AIDS in Uganda. Retrieved from http://www.un.org/esa/population/publications/prospect sdecline/ntozi.pdf.

Ntozi, J. P. M. (2007). *A Review of Research on Older Persons in Uganda.* Prepared for the First East African Policy-Research Diologue on Ageing: Identifying and Addressing Key Information Gaps. *Nairobi.*

OHCHR (2013). Promotion of human rights of older persons in Uganda. Retrieved from http://www.ohchr.org/Documents/Issues/OlderPersons/PublicConsultation2013/UgandaCommissione.

Population Secretariat (2013). *State of Uganda Population Report (2013).* Retrieved from http://countryoffice.unfpa.org/uganda/drive/SUPRE-REPORT-2013lowres.pdf.

Quinn, N. and Knifton, L. (2014). Beliefs, stigma and discrimination associated with mental health problems in Uganda: Implications for theory and practice. *International Journal of Social Psychiatry,* 60(6), 554-561.

Reugg, R.G, Zisook S. and Swerdlow, N. R. (1988). Depression in the aged: an overview. *Psychiatric Clinics of North America, 11*, 83 -99.

Scholten, F., Kinyada, E., Mugisha, J., Seeley, J., Levin, J., Kiwanuka, S. N., … Grosskurth, H. (2010). *Direct and indirect effects of HIV on the health and well being among older people in Uganda.* Prepared for the WHO SAGE Ageing and Health meeting, June 2010. Retrieved from http://www.who.int/healthinfo/14_SAGEcaregiving_Kinyanda.pdf.

Scholten, F., Mugisha, J., Seeley, J., Kinyanda, E., Nakubukwa, S., Kowal, P., Naidoo, N., et al. (2011). Health and functional status among older people with HIV/AIDS in Uganda. *BMC Public Health, 11.*

Seely, J., Zalwango, F., Mugisha, J., Kinyanda, E., Wake, C. and Scholten, F. (2010). *Poverty, aging and HIV/AIDS in Wakiso district.* Paper presented at the Ten Years of 'War Against Poverty': what have we learned since 2000 and what should we do 2010-

2020?, Manchester, UK. Retrieved from http://www.chronicpoverty.org/uploads/publication_files/seeley_et_al_ageing_hiv.pdf.

Seeley, J., Kabunga, E., Tumwekwase, G., Wolff, B. and Grosskurth, H. (2008): The Impact of the AIDS Epidemic on the Lives of Older People in Rural Uganda (Working Paper No. 4). Retrieved from https://www.academia.edu/.

Seeley, J., Wolff, B., Kabunga, E., Tumwekwase, G. and Grosskurth, H. (2009). This is where we buried our sons': people of advanced old age coping with the impact of the AIDS epidemic in a resource-poor setting in rural Uganda. *Ageing and Society, 29*(1), 115-134.

Ssengonzi, R (2007). The plight of older persons as caregivers to people infected/affected by HIV/AIDS: evidence from Uganda. *Journal of Cross-Cultural Gerontology*, *22*(4), 339–353.

Unutzer, J., Katon, W. and Williams, J. W. (2003). Depression Treatment in a sample of 1,801 Depressed Older Adults in Primary Health Care. *Journal of the American Geriatrics Society, 51*(4), 505-514.

Uganda Bureau of Statistics (2014). Uganda National Household Survey (2012/13). Retrieved from http://www.ubos.org/.

Uganda Rural Elderly Support (n.d.). *Background.* Retrieved from http://www.ugres.org/.

Uganda Reach the Aged Association (2009). *Advocacy and the older persons in Uganda.* Retrieved from www.globalgiving.org/pfil/114/projdoc.doc/.

World Federation for Mental Health (2014). Caregivers and mental illness: living with schizophrenia. Retrieved from http://wfmh.com/wp-content/uploads/2014/12/Caregivers-and-Mental-Illness.pdf.

Zimmer, Z. and Dayton, J. (2005). Older adults in sub Saharan Africa living with children and grandchildren. *Population studies, 59*, 295-312.

In: Ageing and Mental Health: Global Perspectives
Editors: Wendy Wen Li, Sherry M. Cummings et al.
ISBN: 978-1-63484-777-3

Chapter 13

CONCLUSION: AGEING AND MENTAL HEALTH IN THE GLOBAL COMMUNITY

Sherry Cummings[1,*], Ilango Ponnuswami[2], Wendy Wen Li[3] and Hong-Jae Park[4]
[1]The University of Tennessee, Knoxville, Tennessee, US
[2]Bharathidasan University, Tiruchirappalli, Tamil Nadu, India
[3]James Cook University, Townsville, Queensland, Australia
[4]The University of Auckland, Auckland, New Zealand

ABSTRACT

To respond to the ageing world, this book sets out to help researchers, policy makers, service providers, and students develop their knowledge of the issues associated with ageing and mental health throughout the world. Written by 21 gerontological experts from Africa, Asia, Europe, North and South America, and Oceania, this book provides an understanding of issues related to ageing and mental health from global perspectives. In this chapter we attempt to integrate the core findings of this book, which reinforce the need for policies and aged care services to respond to the diversity in mental health services for older people in socially, culturally, and geographically different settings. The themes highlighted in this chapter have important implications for policy making, service provision, and the conduct of gerontological research.

Keywords: global perspective, mental health, aged care, policy, services

The worldwide population of older adults is growing at an unprecedented rate. In countries across the globe, the proportion of older adults is rapidly expanding faster than all other age groups. This historic demographic shift heralds momentous transitions in the issues confronting contemporary society. While older adults bring a wealth of wisdom and experience that benefit society, they also possess greater vulnerabilities that present

* Corresponding author: Sherry Cummings, the University of Tennessee. Email: scumming@utk.edu.

substantial societal challenges. The status of mental health disorders among older adults, and individual countries' responses to these disorders, represents one of the greatest of these challenges.

While the worldwide geriatric population is expected to more than triple to 1.5 billion by mid-century, how countries around the globe view and are responding to this phenomenon varies dramatically (National Institute of Ageing [NIA], 2012). More developed countries with greater resources are better able to respond to the health and mental health needs of their elders. Less developed and poorer resourced countries frequently have little ability to investigate and address the needs of their older citizens. In addition to financial resources, countries' responses to older citizens are also influenced by the current numbers of older adults living within their borders and by the views of ageing and older adults that shape the societal consciousness. The chapters in this book represent the global reality of countries that possess great economic diversity, varying proportions of older adults, and differing perspectives on ageing and older adults.

Context and Culture of Ageing and Mental Health

In the previous century attitudes toward older adults were split between a more western and negative view of ageing and an eastern, or traditional, view of ageing that honours elders. Western views of ageing have been shaped by industrialisation and the urbanisation of the population that occurred in the late nineteenth and twentieth centuries. In these societies, such as the U. S., greater value has been attributed to youth who moved in large numbers to cities and produced their own wealth. No longer dependent upon their elders for familial land or power, ties to their older family became more tenuous and support weakened. At the same time, in industrial societies, older adults have been seen as less productive and, therefore, as having less value. The eastern practice of filial piety, and tribal traditions in many countries, upheld the worth and contributions of older adults and the custom of providing care for older family members. Older adults were revered for their wisdom and experience and most often lived in inter-generational family settings that provided for their practical, emotional, and physical needs. However, during the latter part of the 20th century, such views and traditions began to erode due to the urbanisation of populations, modernisation of societies, and the unprecedented ageing process experienced by a broad range of countries from China and Japan to Uganda. Elders' increasing isolation in rural areas in the wake of younger adults' move to urban centers has begun to undermine the traditional system of providing support for older family members, and older family members have progressively come to be viewed as a drain on family resources. Thus, as the global population of elders continues to rapidly expand, worldwide attitudes toward older adults are becoming increasingly more negative.

Stigma related to mental health disorders is also prevalent worldwide. Although the degree of this stigma varies from country to country, mental health disorders are often considered to be a result of personal weakness that brings shame on the individual and, in some cultures, on entire families. Older adults, therefore, are often reluctant to bring mental health issues to the attention of family members and professionals. Furthermore, certain disorders such as depression and dementia are commonly considered by the general populace, family members, professionals and even elders themselves, to be a normal part of ageing and, therefore, not in need of treatment. This combination of ageist attitudes and mental health stigma serves to inhibit the expenditure of funds for the development of programs to address late-life mental health disorders and creates formidable barriers to the access of services, where they do exist, by older adults.

PREVALENCE OF MENTAL HEALTH DISORDERS IN LATER-LIFE

The World Health Organization (2015) has highlighted the prevalence of late-life mental health disorders and the challenges that these present to both individuals and societies. Older adults with psychological and neurological disorders have lower quality of life, increased functional impairment, and higher rates of morbidity and mortality compared to their healthier counterparts. Depressed older adults, for example, suffer from higher percentages of chronic medical illnesses such as diabetes, hypertension, and heart disease (Gildengers, et al., 2013). Significant social and economic burdens related to late-life mental disorders also exist in terms of increased strain on families, and higher medical costs for societies. Chapter authors report that 2% to 10% of older adults within their borders experience dementia, and that that up to 25% struggle with depression. In spite of this, authors also note that both dementia and depression are "silent epidemics" and that high rates of these disorders go undetected. The International Alzheimer's Association (2015) estimates that 46.8 million individuals have dementia and that this number is projected to double in 20 years. Currently, the global economic cost of dementia is US$818 billion. The majority of those with Alzheimer's and related dementias live in developing countries. Furthermore, in coming decades, the most dramatic rise in dementia prevalence is expected to occur in low and middle income countries that are the least prepared to deal with this growing epidemic (Yasamy, Dua, Harper and Saxena, 2013). In order to avoid wide scale suffering, a global response is required to enhance ongoing efforts to find a cure for Alzheimer's Disease and provide needed services to afflicted individuals and families.

Depression is a leading cause of disability and a major contributor to healthcare costs worldwide, yet epidemiological data is not available for many developing countries (Rodda, Walker and Cater, 2011). Experts indicate that worldwide lifetime prevalence is close to 15% (Bromet et al., 2011). Research data from individual countries presented in this book indicate that the prevalence rate of depression among community-based older adults ranges from 11-23%. While few epidemiological studies have been conducted on minor depression, U.S. studies examining this issue indicate that up to 25% of older adults suffer from this disorder, which like major depression is associated with increased medical disorders and mortality (Zarit and Zarit, 2007). Research among institutionalised elders further indicates that up to 28% have been diagnosed with depression and 73% suffer from depressive symptoms (Kaeser, 2012; Pimentel, Afonso and Pereira, 2012). Some factors associated with late-life depression are cross-cultural. Worldwide, women and those who have lost a partner have higher rates of depression. Data varies, however, concerning the contribution of advanced age. In moderate to high-income countries research indicates a diminishment in depression with increased age. However, the reverse appears to be true in less developed countries were a strong positive correlation exists between advancing age and depression (Bromet et al., 2011). This diverging trend may be related to the personal and social resources available to elders in various parts of the globe. In some countries, such as Switzerland, Australia, Hong Kong, Korea, Japan, and the U.S., governments have assumed greater responsibility for the economic and medical needs of their citizens. Other countries, however, do not have the resources to provide such support. In countries such as the U.S. and New Zealand, older adults comprise the group with the lowest poverty rate; in other countries, however, older members represent the poorest segment of the population. In Portugal and Korea for example, 30% and 45% of the older population, respectively, is poor. The plight of large segments of older adults in China and Uganda is also characterised by poverty. Poverty, isolation, and diminished health all contribute to poor mental health among older adults.

Multiple chapter authors, including those from Australia, China, Hong Kong, Japan, Portugal, Switzerland, and the U.S, also reported on the issue of suicide among older adults. All consistently noted that older adults have the highest suicide rate of any population group in their countries. Many countries, however, do not collect such data and so the true pervasiveness of late-life suicide throughout the globe remains unknown. Older adults who suffer from depression, those over 75 years of age, elders living in rural areas and older males have the greatest risk of suicide. Studies indicate that even when older adults have access to, and utilise, medical health services, depressive symptoms and suicidal ideation are often overlooked (Louma, Martin and Pearson, 2002). Clearly, increased education is required for the general population and for health and mental health care practitioners concerning late-life suicide and methods of detecting and effectively responding to symptoms.

Little data is available regarding the prevalence of other mental health disorders among older adults across the globe. Some data does exist concerning late-life anxiety; however, differences between countries are present. In the U.S. and Australia, for example, anxiety disorders are present in up to 10% of older individuals. Older Koreans, on the other hand, have lower rates of anxiety disorders than do their western counterparts. Information concerning late–life substance abuse, although limited, is increasingly coming to the fore. Alcohol abuse, prescription drug misuse and, in some cultures, illegal drugs, are becoming more prevalent. In Australia, for example, older adults have the highest number of deaths related to psychoactive drugs while alcohol abuse is one of the most common mental health disorders among older Portuguese. In both the U.S. and Switzerland approximately 6% of the older population misuse or abuse alcohol. As noted by multiple authors, the proportion of older adults with substance abuse problems is expected to increase as the number of older baby boomers around the globe continues to grow. For this reason, experts predict that the demand for effective treatments for older adults who misuse substances will dramatically escalate in coming years (Gfroerer, Penne, Pemberton and Folsom, 2003).

Data concerning severe mental illnesses (SMI) among older adults is limited worldwide. Research suggests that in the U.S. alone over one million older adults have some type of severe psychological disorder. Elders with severe mental disorders typically have higher levels of functional impairment, fewer resources, poorer physical health, and require more care from family members and the community (Awad and Voruganti, 2008). In spite of this, little is known about these elders and the needs of their family members. Those with SMI have shorter lifespans and in some countries smaller percentages of those with the disorders reach later life. Because of the bizarre nature of some symptoms, such as hallucinations and delusions, greater stigma is also attached to these disorders. In addition, different cultures have divergent interpretations of psychotic behavior and, therefore, what is classified as a severe mental illness in one culture may not be the same as such classifications in other cultures. This subsequently inhibits the development of knowledge concerning the number of older adults across the globe who suffer from SMI and the delivery of effective treatment.

SERVICES FOR OLDER ADULTS WITH MENTAL HEALTH DISORDERS

The type and extent of mental health services for older adults across the globe varies greatly not only from country to country, but also, within countries. These services are administered by a variety of entities within individual countries including national and state agencies, non-governmental/non-profit organisations, and churches. They fall under the auspices of multiple systems including health, mental health, and social service. Because of these differences and variations, the true nature and extent of the mental health services extended to the elderly is difficult to discern. In general, the services available for older adults throughout the world are less developed and widespread than are services that exist for those who are younger. In some more highly developed countries a variety of gero-psychiatric services are available. These range from hospital and residential to community and home-based programs. Specialised in-patient psychogeriatric units, community psychiatric teams, dementia care programs, both daily and residential, community mental health centers with services such as outreach, casework counselling, support groups, social and recreational programs, and nursing homes do exist, in varying degrees, in countries such as Australia, Hong Kong, Korea, New Zealand, Switzerland and the U.S. These programs deliver critical assistance to older adults experiencing acute psychiatric episodes, supportive services to those with on-going mental health issues living in the community, residential care for those unable to live on their own, and needed help to family members providing care. Not all of these services are provided in all developed countries and most chapter authors note that some of the services that do exist in their countries are less available in certain regions and in rural areas. As can be seen from earlier chapters, in more developed countries efforts are underway to maintain older adults with mental health needs in the community through the provision of an array of supportive mental services.

Remaining in the home is a goal of most older adults, including those struggling with dementia, depression, and other psychiatric disorders. However, the symptoms and consequences of these disorders, coupled with physical illnesses and functional impairments that are common in later life, can present formidable challenges to ageing in place. As families become increasingly geographically splintered, their ability to provide needed care for older members with mental health disorders deteriorates. In low to moderately developed countries that do not posses an integrated system of support for older citizens, when families are unavailable or overtaxed, assistance, if available, is found primarily in hospitals or nursing homes. In the least developed countries, such as Uganda, that are struggling to meet the basic health care needs of their citizens, older adults have even less access to the limited health facilities than do others. Elders in dire need of mental health care, at times, may find temporary treatment in general in-patient units. Thus, in high-income countries with more advanced health and mental health care, a system of mental health services for older adults is being developed, although notable gaps often persist. In moderate and low-income countries, few, and at times, no specialised mental health services are available.

Various studies also indicate a high prevalence of mental illness in nursing homes. Dementia and depression appear to be the most common mental disorders in this setting. However, most residents with mental disorders do not receive adequate treatment. Barriers to good treatment include: (1) a shortage of specialised mental health professionals trained in geriatrics; (2) lack of knowledge and inadequate training of nursing home staff about mental health issues; (3) lack of public financial reimbursements to facilities for the coverage of behavioural and mental health problems; and (4) difficulty obtaining the services of psychiatrists and other mental health professionals due to inadequate reimbursement policies. Thus, there is a great need to incorporate mental health care into the basic structure of nursing home care and to make professional services available to patients and their families. In the end, an appropriate and supportive legislative environment based on internationally accepted human rights standards is required to ensure the highest quality of community and residential based services to people with mental illness and their caregivers (WHO, 2015).

CAREGIVING

The World Health Organization (2011) notes the crucial contribution that family members make in providing care to older family members. Multiple social, psychological, and biological factors determine the level of mental and physical health of a person at any point of time. Due to these factors as well as the typical life stressors common to all people, many older adults lose their ability to live independently and require some form of on-going care. In addition, older people are more likely to experience events such as bereavement, a drop in socioeconomic status with retirement, or a disability. All of these factors can result in isolation, loss of independence, loneliness, and psychological distress in older people (WHO, 2015). Caregiving assumes a prominent role in the field of gerontology and geriatrics with an increasingly greater proportion of older persons requiring different types of care. Older persons suffering from physical and mental health problems, in addition to, enormous economic and psychosocial difficulties, are in need of a variety of services by care professionals and informal carers.

As evidenced by information presented in this book, the rapid expansion of the older population has led to a dramatic increase in the demand experienced by families throughout the world to provide care to their older members. Although developed countries have witnessed a decline in intergenerational households for multiple decades, primary caregivers for older adults in these countries continue to be family members. Chapter authors from Australia and the U.S., for example, note, that 75% and 85%, respectively, of all care provided to older adult in these two countries comes from family members. Further, chapter authors from Hong Kong, Portugal, and Korea echo the claim that families continue to provide the majority of care for older members. In more developed countries, familial caregivers receive varying degrees of governmental assistance. In Hong Kong, for example, community-based services are provided to support caregivers in social service settings. The Swiss government provides some economic assistance for caregivers through their Mandatory Basic Health Insurance Program. In other countries various services such as psycho-educational support, counselling, and adult day cares are available to caregivers of older adults. It should be noted that in many cases such services are primarily focused on providing aid to dementia caregivers. Supports for informal carers of elders with other types of mental health disorders is often less available.

In less developed countries where poverty is rampant, and there is little to no safety net for people as they age, older adults' lack of financial resources and the shortage of governmental supports create an even greater demand on families to assume care. This situation is exacerbated in countries such as such as India and Uganda where state provided supports and services for caregivers are very scarce, and in some regions of the country, non-existent. Consequently, the full physical, emotional, and economic burden of providing care to older members falls directly on resource-deprived and economically struggling families. As reported by the chapter authors for these two countries, the above factors can lead to tragic consequences such as elder abuse and abandonment.

Women throughout the globe, from the most to the least developed countries, assume the main responsibility for providing informal care to the older generation. In addition to providing the majority of assistance, women are also more likely to administer hands-on care such as dressing, bathing and preparing food for elder family members (National Alliance for Caregiving, 2009). In the U.S. over 60% of familial caregivers are female. In South Korea the daughter-in-law is expected to assume primary responsibility for caregiving activities. Women who provide care must often reduce work hours or abandon employment to fulfill their caregiving responsibilities. As a result, these women may lose the opportunity for advancement in the work place and experience a decrease in pensions received when such opportunities are available (Lahaie, Earle and Heymann, 2012). Older adults, who are often struggling with their own medical and functional issues, also frequently assume caregiving responsibilities for an impaired spouse. In Australia and the U.S. 20% of all caregivers are spouses/partners aged 65 and over, while in Hong Kong 26.3%, and in Switzerland a full third, are spouses, with most of these caregivers being wives. Women have long held main caregiving responsibilities for families. However, due to the dwindling size of families across the globe fewer women are now available to provide care for the rapidly growing number of older adults who are living longer lives with greater impairments. In order to maintain the health and functioning of families throughout the world, it is necessary that governments affirm the value of older impaired members of society and provide the supports needed by families so that they may effectively provide for their elders' care.

POLICIES

Policies exist in countries throughout the world that support the health and well-being of older adults. In rare instances nations have established policies and laws that directly target the treatment of mental disorders and the promotion of mental well-being among older citizens. New Zealand's Positive Ageing Strategy, which is the country's main initiative for the implementation of older adult social services and programs and which is aligned with national efforts to promote positive aging, is such an example. Likewise, in 1997 Australia passed the Aged Care Act that led to the development of a national mental health strategy and a national respite program for caregivers.

In most countries, however, a variety of policies exist that focus on some aspect of older adult well-being and on mental health for the general population. These combined policies offer varying degrees of support for older adult services and, at times, for older adult mental health. For example in Japan, the national government implemented policy, *Long-Term Care*, is a nationally mandated long-term care insurance programme for older adults that includes universal coverage for pensions, health insurance, and long-term care. While this programme does not specifically focus on mental health, the services that it supports have made it possible for Japanese citizens to live longer healthier lives. In addition, in 2002 the Japanese government developed a community mental health care program that benefits all citizens, including elders, by shifting the focus of mental health care from hospital-based medical treatment to community-centred care. In the United States Medicare, a universal health insurance program for those 65 years of age and older, addresses acute health and mental health care needs of older adults. This policy, however, does not include all older adults nor cover all mental health services. Another program, Medicaid, extends coverage to low-income individuals including children, pregnant women, persons with disabilities, and older adults, and targets both acute and long-term care needs.

Other countries have not enacted policies and programmes that focus specifically on older adults, but do have legislation and related services that benefit older citizens. In Korea, for example, social insurance, public assistance, and social welfare programs provide health, financial, and practical assistance. Although these policies and services do not explicitly target older adults with mental health needs, they do offer some help or care for older citizens. Similarly, while there is no specific elderly mental health policy in Hong Kong, differing aspects of older adult mental health services are subsumed under the country's medical and social service systems. A national bureau has overall responsibility for coordinating the various mental health service programs. The Portuguese *National Health Plan* does not focus specifically on older adults; however, this plan does promote strategies that positively impact the older population, including an increase in mental health services, improvement in community-based mental health care, and implementation of mental health related prevention and promotion programmes. In Switzerland, health and long-term care are de-centralised and under the control of three different levels of government from federal to local. The Swiss Health Observatory, which has a branch that focuses on mental health, and the Swiss Mental Health Network were both created within the past 15 years and have heightened focus on mental health, especially mental health and working life. While most older adults are not currently employed, these efforts to support mental health in Switzerland do benefit older citizens.

Some countries have national policies targeting older adults that posses varying foci and depth. For example, the Chinese government enacted a law in 2012 entitled *Protection of the Rights and Interests of Elderly People* that outlined the duties of children as they relate to their older parents, including the obligation to be concerned about older family members' mental health. In India, the well-being of older citizens is mandated in the Constitution, and the *National Programme for the Health Care of the Elderly* contains provisions for welfare services, while the Ugandan Constitution recognizes the value and rights of the elderly and stipulates that the government make "reasonable provision for the welfare and maintenance" of older adults. These measures highlight the governments' recognition of the importance, and needs, of their older citizens. They do not, however, provide for funding or the establishment of specific services to meet older adults' health and mental health care needs.

As can be seen, extant national policies that directly target older adult mental health are uncommon. Among countries that do provide some type of mental health services for older adults, more common approaches include coverage of older adults under policies created for general populations and/or coverage provision through a variety of health, financial, and welfare services. While older adults do benefit from these policies and programmes, such approaches often provide insufficient services and contain gaps in coverage. Services focused on general populations often do not possess the necessary elements for effective management of older adults. Transportation, accessible settings, and the presence of personnel with geriatric knowledge are all essential for the effective care and treatment of older adults. These are often lacking in non-specialised programme and service settings. On the other hand, programs and services that are designed for older adults but are created under, and directed by, separate policies often possess differing goals and approaches. As a result, a lack of communication and coordination among mental health, health and ageing programmes is prevalent and gaps in essential services occur (Cummings and Kropf, 2011). Less developed nations often focus scarce resources on the basic needs of their citizens. While the plight of their older citizens is recognised, they do not posses the means or infrastructure to develop and operate services focused on older adult care.

Gaps in Mental Health Aged Care and Recommendations

To analyse the gaps in mental health services for older persons, it is necessary to first consider the overall mental health scenario of the world. According to the Mental Health Atlas (WHO, 2014), just 68% of WHO Member States have a stand-alone policy or plan for mental health and 51% have a stand-alone mental health law. In addition, levels of public expenditures on mental health are very low even in low and middle-income countries, less than US$2 per capita (WHO, 2014). These data evidence a world community still struggling with recognition of the deleterious impact of mental health disorders on individuals and societies. Within this context, the mental health needs of older adults are often obscured. However, given the rapid, inexorable growth of the older adult population worldwide and the high prevalence of dementias, depression, and other mental health disorders among this population, urgent attention to older adult mental health is needed to avoid unnecessary suffering among older individuals, increased burden among familial caregivers, and heightened negative social and economic impacts among nations.

The country-focused chapters of this volume have brought to light important features of elder care across the globe. Large numbers of elderly individuals neither seek nor receive effective mental health treatment. Chapter authors discussed numerous barriers to treatment. Ageist attitudes, which are prevalent throughout the world, hinder the recognition of need for treatment by family members, professionals and older adults themselves. Mental health stigma and illiteracy are also prevalent. Limited knowledge and understanding of the nature of and treatment for mental health problems was cited a major factor in low and inappropriate treatment seeking among older individuals with mental health problems. A common theme in multiple chapters was the shortage of professionals with specialised geriatric training. In spite of growing need, the education of geriatric health professionals across the globe falls far short of stated demand. This shortage results in limited awareness of, and attention to, older adults' mental health needs, mis- and under-diagnosis of late-life mental health disorders, and inadequate development of geriatric mental health services. Countries throughout the world must develop strategies to rapidly expand the ranks of health and mental health professionals competently prepared to work with older adults and their families. Efforts in these areas are critical to meeting the predictable demands of the burgeoning older population. Public education programs in nations throughout the globe are also urgently needed to inform the general population and policy makers of the gifts that healthy ageing confers to individuals and societies, the characteristics of mental health disorders that all too often destroy late-life potential, and the effective interventions that currently exist to treat mental health disorders in later life.

Overall, WHO (2015) reports that approximately 20% of older adults worldwide suffer from neurological and psychological disorders. This is an estimate that suggests the magnitude of the problem facing the global community. However, the true prevalence remains unknown. In order for the worldwide community and individual countries to effectively respond to the mental health challenges faced by their older citizens it is necessary that, as a first step, they have the ability and the resources to detect later-life mental health disorders. As can been seen from the chapters in this book, challenges exist in determining the true prevalence of late-life mental health disorders. Many countries lack national studies examining the types and prevalence of mental health disorders among their older citizens. The author of the chapter on Switzerland, for example, noted that comprehensive national data on mental disorder prevalence does not exist for that country and that very little information is available concerning older adults. In some countries, such as India and China, small local and regional studies have been conducted that provide some data. In other countries, such as Uganda scant information exits about mental health status of older adults. Systematic research and epidemiological studies are needed so that countries have an accurate understanding of the nature and characteristics of their growing older population, and that meaningful polices may be developed to address older adult s' mental health needs.

Mental health services for older adults vary significantly across the globe, and inadequate systems of care are common. Upon reviewing the prevalence of psychological and neurological disorders worldwide and extant mental health care systems, the WHO (2013) urged the adoption of two specific service strategies. First recommended was the systematic shift of locus of care away from long-stay mental hospitals toward service provided by a network of linked community-based mental health services. Such services include comprehensive mental health centers, primary care, short-term inpatient, day care centers, and support of people with mental disorders living with their families. The second recommended strategy was the establishment of integrated and coordinated care systems that focuses on holistic prevention, promotion and rehabilitation, and that address both mental and physical health care needs.

Dr. Margaret Chan, Director General of the World Health Organization, in her Foreword to the mpGAP Intervention Guide Version 1.0, stated:

> Health systems around the world face enormous challenges in delivering care and protecting the human rights of people with mental, neurological and substance use disorders. The resources available are insufficient, inequitably distributed and inefficiently used. As a result, a large majority of people with these disorders receives no care at all (WHO, 2010).

Good general health and social care is important for promoting older people's health, preventing disease, and managing chronic illnesses. Training all health providers in working with issues and disorders related to ageing is therefore important. Effective, community-level primary mental health care for older people is crucial. It is equally important to focus on the long-term care of older adults suffering from mental disorders, as well as to provide caregivers with education, training, and support. Older adults throughout the world are a valuable resource to the global community; but, it is up to global, national and local leaders to recognise the challenges that this population faces, and through sustained commitment work together to develop systems and strategies that promote the mental and physical well-being of the ever growing numbers of elderly though out the world.

CONCLUSION

Obviously, the face of the global population is changing. Countries across the world are experiencing unprecedented ageing of their populations, and with that, increased prevalence of mental illness. This reality puts substantial strain on health care systems and requires governments and policy makers to respond with thorough and effective support systems. It is necessary to change social perceptions about ageing with regard to stereotypes as well as what is considered normal ageing. To achieve this, the priority is to conduct further research into the prevalence of mental illness among older people, as well as to investigate the developing needs of this population. This would enable the relevant parties to provide improved education and support. The future for most countries across the world will be challenging, but hopefully these challenges will be met with research, support, and improved care systems for older people with mental illness, providing a positive outlook as we move forward.

REFERENCES

Awad, A. G. and Voruganti, L. (2008). The burden of schizophrenia on caregivers. *Pharmaco Economics, 26*, 149-162.

Bromet, E., Andrade, L. H. Hwang, I., Sampson, N. A., Alonso, J. and de Girolamo, G. (2011). Cross-national epidemiology of DSM-IV major depressive episode. *BMC Medicine, 9,* 90.

Cummings, S. M. and Kropf, N. P. (2011). Aging with a Severe Mental Illness: Challenges and Treatments. *Journal of Gerontological Social Work, 54, 175-188.*

Gildengers, A., Tatsuoka, C., Bialko, C., Cassidy, K. A., Dines, P., Emanuel, J., … Sajatoovic, M.S. (2013). Correlates of disability in depressed older adults with bipolar disorder. *Cut Edge Psychiatry Practice, 1*, 332-338.

Gfroerer, J., Penne, M., Pemberton, M. and Folsom, R. (2003). Substance abuse treatment needs among older adults in 2020: the impact of the aging baby-boom cohort. *Drug and Alcohol Dependence, 29*, 127-135.

International Alzheimer's Association. (2015). *World Alzheimer's report 2105, the global impact of dementia: An analysis of prevalence, incidence, cost and trends.* London: Alzheimer's Disease International.

Kaeser, M. (2012). *Santé des personnes âgées vivant en établissement médico-social. Enquête sur la santé des personnes âgées dans les institutions 2008/09* [Health of old persons living in nursing homes. Swiss Survey on Old People Living in Institution 2008/09]. Neuchâtel: OFS.

Lahaie, C., Earle, A. and Heymann, J. (2012). An Uneven Burden: Social Disparities in Adult Caregiving Responsibilities, Working Conditions, and Caregiver Outcomes. *Research on Aging, 35*, 243-274.

Louma, J. B., Martin, C. E. and Pearson, J. L. (2002). Contact with mental health and primary care providers before suicide: A review of evidence. *American Journal of Psychiatry, 159*, 909-916.

National Alliance for Caregiving. (2009). Executive summary: Caregiving in the U.S. Retrieved from http://www.caregiving.org/pdf/research/CaregivingUSAllAgesExec Sum.pdf.

National Institute on Aging (2012). National Institutes of Health. NIH publication # - 11-7737. Global Health and Aging.

Pimentel, A. F., Afonso, R. M and Pereira, H. (2012). Depression and support in old age. *Psicologia, Saúde and Doenças, 13(2),* 311-327.

Rodda, J., Walker, Z. and Cater, J. (2011). Depression in older adults. *BMJ.* 343:d5219 doi: 10.1136/bmj.d5219.

WHO (2010). mhGap intervention guide for mental, neurological and substance use disorders in non-specialized health settings. Mental Health Gap Action Programme.

WHO (2011). *Global health and aging*. National Institutes on Aging and National Institute of Health. NIH Publication no. 11-7737.

WHO. (2013). Comprehensive mental health action plan 2013–2020. Retrieved from http://www.who.int/mental_health/publications/action_plan/e n/.

WHO (2015), *Mental health and older adults,* Fact Sheet No.381, September. Retrieved from http://www.who.int/mediacentre/factsheets/fs381/en/.

Yasamy, M.T., Dua, T., Harper, M., Saxena, S. (2013). Mental health of older adults: Addressing a growing concern. *World Health Organization*, Department of Mental Health and Substance Abuse.

Zarit, S. H. and Zarit, J. M. (2007). *Mental Disorders in Older Adults: Fundamentals of Assessment and Treatment.* New York, NY: The Gildford Press.

ABOUT THE CONTRIBUTORS

Dr. Carole Adamson is currently a senior social work lecturer at the University of Auckland, where her research and teaching focuses on mental health, trauma, resilience and stress. She has research interests in developing resilient practitioners and in social work curriculum for disaster preparation and response. She has been a mental health social worker in acute and forensic settings, and also has experience in community development and residential social work. She sees a major focal point in her work as the articulation of theoretical perspectives and frameworks for social work practice that can integrate current, contextually-aware best practice and which can effectively be applied in practice settings.

Dr. Alma Au is the Research Coordinator of the Institute of Active Ageing at Hong Kong Polytechnic University. She works as Associate Professor at the Department of Applied Social Sciences at the University and is the Director of the Child Development Centre. She is also a Visiting Fellow of The Oxford Institute of Population Ageing. She was initially trained in psychology and is a Fellow of the Hong Kong Psychological Society. She has practiced clinical psychology both with the National Health Service in London and the Hospital Authority in Hong Kong. After moving to the University, she has obtained a number of grants both from both local and international government and non-government organizations to develop community-based assessments and interventions. She has published in various international journals. Her current interests include developing sustainable models of health care and active aging in the context of inter-generational relationships.

Dr. Xue Bai is Assistant Professor in the Department of Applied Social Sciences at Hong Kong Polytechnic University. She also serves as visiting fellow at Personal Social Services Research Unit in London School of Economics and Political Science, honorary research fellow at Sau Po Centre on Ageing in the University of Hong Kong, and honorary research consultant at Jockey Club Centre for Positive Ageing. Her areas of research and teaching mainly include ageing and health, active ageing, retirement and long-term care issues. Dr. Bai has been trying to connect research to practice, using research to inform service provision in different local NGOs through program assessments and evaluations. Her work has been widely published in renowned international journals in the above-mentioned research areas.

Dr. Wai-chi Chan is a Clinical Associate Professor of Department of Psychiatry, The University of Hong Kong. He is also the Honorary Consultant and Head of Psychogeriatric

Services at Queen Mary Hospital in Hong Kong. Dr. Chan is currently the Chief Editor of the East Asian Archives of Psychiatry, and the Vice President of the Chinese Dementia Research Association. In addition, he is a member of the Working Group on Active Ageing under the Elderly Commission, and an advisor to various non-governmental organisations. His research interests include cognitive disorders, depression and psychiatric epidemiology.

Yan Chen is a full-time doctoral student in School of Educational Sciences and Psychology at University of Eastern Finland (UEF). She was awarded her Masters degree in psychological counseling at China University of Geosciences. She currently devotes herself to the study of family psychology/therapy and research of family changes post suicide in China, while completing her PhD at UEF.

Dr. Sherry Cummings is professor and Associate Dean for the University of Tennessee, College of Social Work (UTCSW) in the United States. She is a fellow of the Gerontological Society of America and past president of the Association of Gerontological Education in Social Work (AGESW). Dr. Cummings' area of research and practice focuses on aging and mental health, in particular, older adults with depression, severe mental illness and alcohol misuse disorders. She has published over 40 articles and two books and presents widely at national and international conferences.

Elizabeth Galleguillos is currently finalising her PhD at the University of Lausanne, where she has worked as a teaching assistant. Awarded by the Swiss National Science Foundation, she spent a year period at the Oxford Institute of Population Ageing (OIPA), where she participated as a research officer in the international LARNA project. In the past, she worked at the Department of Political Science/Resop at University of Geneva, where she held a position of research office, and at the Institute of Political, Historical and International Studies (IEPHI) of the University of Lausanne as a teaching assistant. She has a particular interest on ageing societies, the role of ideology and their implications for states arrangements.

Dr. Xuewei Huang is a professor of psychiatry, the Director of the department of psychiatry and medical psychology, and part of the clinical medicine college at Guangdong Pharmaceutical University. Her research focuses on psychotherapy and its application, especially on cancer care. She has made significant contributions to psychotherapy and its theory and methods. She has received awards for both her teaching and one of her books. Throughout her career, Professor Huang has published 6 books and more than 40 journal articles.

Dr. Sofia von Humboldt is a clinical and health psychologist with a long-standing experience with older adults. She has been principal investigator on grants from the Portuguese Foundation for Science and Technology. Her current research and scholarly interests include adjustment to aging, mental health, personhood in dementia and psychosis, sexual well-being, health care and cross-cultural studies with older populations. Dr. von Humboldt is Associate Professor and Principal Investigator in William James Research Center at ISPA-Instituto Universitário de Ciências Psicológicas, Sociais e da Vida. Deeply committed to working with older adults, she has written papers, chapters and books on the distinctive multidimensional and cross-cultural approach to mental health in old age.

Kassandra Jackson completed her psychology degree at James Cook University in 2013, during which she produced a thesis and participated in the Unity in Diversity conference. Since then, she has been involved in a number of research projects focusing on ageing and mental health in the tropics, as well as in the production of a number of book chapters with an ageing and mental health focus. Presently, she is working to complete her Masters while developing teaching skills through lecturing and tutoring Intercultural and Social Psychology subjects. Kassandra is the Assistant Editor of this book.

Dr. Hiroko Kase is a professor of gerontology at Waseda University, Japan. She received her M.A. (Social Welfare Program) from Japan Women's University, and was appointed as a community social worker working with the elderly at Musashino city. After her seven-year career as a community social worker, she was offered tenure at the Japan College of Social Work. Her research interest is the policy and methodology of elderly care. Subsequently, she received her Ph.D. from Waseda University for a dissertation titled: Analysis and Evaluation of Care Management Focusing on Behavioral and Psychological Symptoms with Dementia. (2013). In addition to teaching, Dr. Kase works for professionals in practice as a supervisor, and is the vice president of the Japan Academy of Home Care. She currently resides in central of Tokyo, where she was born and raised, with her husband.

Dr. Dongbae Kim graduated from the University of Michigan, Ann Arbor, Michigan, in the United States, in 1988. He received a Master in Social Work and a Ph. D. in Urban and Regional Planning. He founded the School of Social Welfare at Yonsei University in 2001, the first of its type in Korea and became the first Dean of the School. He has taught and written in the areas of Welfare for Older Adults, Voluntarism, Christian Social Work, and recently Spirituality and Social Work. He became a professor emeritus in 2015.

Dr. Betty Kyaddondo is a senior medical doctor in the field of demography and public health. She previously coordinated the African Youth Alliance Project under Kampala City Council and served as a Medical Coordinator for AIDS Information Centre (AIC). She currently heads the Family Health Department (FHD) at Population Secretariat responsible for national population policy development, management and coordination. She also coordinates the Partners in Population and Development for Uganda. She affiliated with Child Health and Development Centre with over 15 years of experience in women and children health research, rights and gender based health research and programming intended to address needs of the most vulnerable and hard to reach sectors of the population including women, children and adolescents for purposes of accelerating the achievement of the Millennium Development Goals. She has worked with policy makers at all levels to put health, population and geriatric issues high on the development agenda. She is a 2014 Collen Fellow for the Oxford Institute of Population Ageing, Oxford University, UK.

Hyo Jung Lee is currently a doctoral candidate in the Department of Gerontology at the McCormack Graduate School of Policy and Global Studies at the University of

Massachusetts, Boston. She received her Master of Science in Gerontology in 2012 from the University of Massachusetts Boston, and Master in Social Work in 2006 from the School of Social Welfare at Yonsei University.

Hongyu Li works at Guangdong Pharmaceutical University as a lecturer. She has a Masters of Science in Medical Psychology and studied at the Institute of Psychology, Chinese Academy of Sciences. Her research focuses on basic psychology and personality psychology, especially on humanistic theory and psychotherapy.

Dr. Wendy Wen Li is a Senior Lecturer in Psychology in College of Healthcare Sciences at James Cook University, Australia. Prior to her current appointment she was a Teaching Fellow in School of Psychology at the University of Waikato, a Counsellor at the Asian Services of the Problem Gambling Foundation of New Zealand, and a Senior Lecturer at Guangdong Women's Polytechnic College in China. Dr. Li is currently a Research Fellow of The Cairns Institute, JCU; an Associate of WHO Collaborating Centres for Nursing and Midwifery Education and Research Capacity Building; a Research Associate with School of Psychology at the University of Waikato, New Zealand; and a Senior Research Consultant for Verité (a US-based NGO) of the China Office. Dr. Li has an extensive research experience and led projects in Australia, New Zealand and China in areas of ageing, mental health, intergroup relations and discrimination, migration and refugee, and problem gambling and substance abuse.

Email: Wendy.Li@jcu.edu.au

Ho-ming Yip is a Research Associate in the Department of Applied Social Sciences of The Hong Kong Polytechnic University. He has obtained a master degree in Social Work and has involved in different local government consultancy projects related to social welfares. He is also involved in different projects providing intervention to dementia caregivers and parents in at-risk families. Currently, Mr. Yip is participating in projects about old adults, by using bottom-up approach and community-based intervention, aiming to make Hong Kong a more age-friendly city.

Dr. Hong-Jae Park is a Senior Lecturer with School of Counselling, Human Services and Social Work, Faculty of Education and Social Work, The University of Auckland. He is a native of South Korea who moved to Aotearoa New Zealand in 2003. He has taught a range of undergraduate and postgraduate courses including ethics and justice, lifespan development, disability research, and applied professional practice in the field of social work and human services. Dr. Park's area of research and practice focuses on migrant and diaspora communities, gerontological concerns (in particular, older people in a foreign land), and mental health in late life. Recently, he has undertaken a series of studies on filial piety and elder abuse across cultures and regions.

Dr. Ilango Ponnuswami is currently Professor and Head, Department of Social Work, Bharathidasan University, Tiruchirappalli, India. With a Fellowship from the UNFPA and the UN International Institute on Ageing, Malta, he successfully pursued a Post Graduate Diploma in Gerontology and Geriatrics at the Institute of Gerontology, University of Malta. He has been actively researching on various aspects of ageing, publishing and presenting papers in national and international ageing conferences. Dr. Ponnuswami represented India at the BRICS Forum on Ageing recently held in Seoul, South Korea.

Shannon M. Trecartin is a PhD Candidate at the University of Tennessee. She is also an Assistant Professor in the Department of Social Work at Andrews University, Michigan. Her area of research is disability and older adults.

Teresa B. K. Tsien is the Professional Consultant and Professor of Practice of the Institute of Active Ageing, Hong Kong Polytechnic University. She is a part-time visiting lecturer for the MSc in Clinical Gerontology programme at the Chinese University of Hong Kong. She specializes in teaching and research on dementia care, carer support, lifelong learning and active ageing. She is a reviewer for the British Journal of Social Work, Hong Kong Social Workers Association Journal, Hong Kong Nursing Journal and HKSAR Central Policy Unit. Teresa was appointed to various public boards by the HKSAR government, such as YauTsimMong South District Committee, Kowloon City Fight Crime Committee, Social Welfare Advisory Committee, Community Chest and Guardianship Board. She serves as President of WINGS HK, Vice Chairman of Senior Citizen Home Safety Association, Hon. Treasurer of the Hong Kong Alzheimer's Disease Association, a member of the Elderly Committee of the Hong Kong Council of Social Service. She also serves as an advisor to eight non-government organizations.

Dr. P. Udhayakumar is currently an Assistant Professor, Department of Social Work, Central University of Tamil Nadu, Thiruvarur, South India. Earlier, he served as a Teaching Assistant at the Bharathidasan University, Tiruchirappalli, South India. He obtained his Masters in Social Work and Ph. D in Social Work form Bharathidasan University, Tiruchirappalli, South India. He is also a Student Counsellor for Counselling and Guidance Cell, Central University of Tamil Nadu. Dr. P. Udhayakumar has published research article in reputed journal like Indian Journal of Gerontology, International Journal of Applied Management and Journal of Research, Extension and Development. He has presented scientific papers at various International and National Conferences conducted by various reputed organisations.

INDEX

D

E

H

I

J

K

L

M

N

O

Q

R

S

Y